Pamela Vass

On Course for Recovery

Boundstone Books

First published in Great Britain in 2013 by
Boundstone Books, Little Boundstone, Littleham,
Bideford. EX39 5HW.

Copyright © Pamela Vass 2013

All rights reserved. No part of this
publication may be reproduced,
transmitted or stored in a retrieval system
in any form or by any means without
permission in writing from
Boundstone Books.

ISBN 978-0-9568709-1-9

Cover image: Clip art
Cover design: Terry Sackett
Printed by: Short Run Press, Exeter

www.boundstonebooks.co.uk

Acknowledgements

My thanks go to Laurence Shelley, Terry Sackett, Jacqui Poole, Shelia Bees, Hilary Jones, the Hartland Writing Group, Rosemary Walters and all those who attended 'Time for Me' courses for their invaluable scrutiny and feedback.

The extracts headed, *'The Fight Between Two Wolves'* and *'Who am I*?' source unknown.

Important

This course should not be viewed as a replacement for any prescribed treatment or medical advice. It is an additional resource for you to consider dependent upon your unique circumstances and to be followed according to your own judgement.

Dedication

This book is dedicated to, and inspired by, the members of MEND (ME North Devon) who attended my courses and whose testimonials and contributions are gratefully acknowledged.

*

'This course made me focus on things that would help me recover.'

'Grasp the opportunity - I feel empowered to carry on with life.'

'Go for it, work at it, enjoy it!'

'Thank you for providing a safe haven where it didn't feel wrong to put myself first for a change.'

'All the information given was enlightening.'

*

'I recommend this course to anyone.'
Rosemary Walter, Chair, ME North Devon

Tutored courses

Introductory courses and workshops based on this text and led by Pamela are available for groups. For further information see: www.boundstonebooks.co.uk

Contents

		Page
Chapter 1	Introduction	6
Chapter 2	How Are You?	10
Chapter 3	Forecasting Your Day	27
Chapter 4	The Power of Choice	41
Chapter 5	Boom and Bust	52
Chapter 6	Choices	68
Chapter 7	Time for some T.L.C.	79
Chapter 8	A Different Language	91
Chapter 9	A Sense of Hope	103
Chapter 10	Rediscovering Your Self	116
Chapter 11	A Picture of Health	125
Postscript	'My Story'	135
Appendix	Suggested Reading	142

Chapter 1

Introduction

You are not alone. Over a quarter of a million people suffer from M.E. or Chronic Fatigue Syndrome in the UK. Many others remain undiagnosed. There is no apparent cure yet it is possible to recover, as I have.

Are you ready to find your road to recovery?

You are not your illness. You are a person with hopes, dreams and a life to live. You may have lost sight of that person but you're there - waiting to be rediscovered.

You've picked up this book and read this far. Now you have a choice. Do you put it down? Or do you decide that you've had enough of struggling with this illness and it's time to set yourself on course for recovery?

'If only,' I hear you say! I felt the same way before I discovered that it *is* possible to influence our own health. Through the simple exercises described in this course, I began to see how.

I thought I was already doing everything possible to

recover, trying all sorts of therapies and taking supplements. They just weren't working. Then I realised that when we hit a crisis such as chronic illness we need to dig deeper, to find new solutions.

This course will help you discover those solutions for yourself. Follow it individually or join with others for support and encouragement. Work on a different chapter each week or stay with each section for a month or more; whatever feels right for you.

Very soon you'll discover how to support your body's natural healing process... and find yourself on course for recovery.

As you follow this course you will:

- identify what drains your energy
- discover what's blocking progress
- learn to listen and respond to your body
- understand how to avoid ups and downs
- begin to play an active part in your recovery

This book focuses on what *you* can do.

Do you dream of feeling well again? Maybe you've tried one practitioner after another hoping the next will hold the secret to your recovery. But therapies that have worked for others may not hold the same benefits for you.

It doesn't have to be this way.

You don't need to feel helpless. There is much you can do to support your body. It may not be functioning as it should, resulting in symptoms with which you are all too familiar, but the body has an amazing ability to self-heal, given the right conditions. This course provides you with the tools to identify and create those conditions for yourself.

This kind of change doesn't come from outside, from the actions of others or a change in circumstances. It comes from within. The emphasis is on *you,* on the positive, effective action **you** can take **right now** to make a difference to your life.

There are a few things you will need. These are:

- ☑ a notebook, preferably attractive, something you value
- ☑ a pen
- ☑ two highlighter pens
- ☑ a bookmark
- ☑ private time

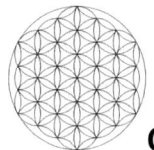

CHAPTER 1 SUMMARY

➥ This book is a course for you to follow, either individually or in a group

➥ Through this course you will learn how to provide the best possible healing environment for your body

➥ This kind of change doesn't come from outside - from the actions of others or a change in circumstances; it comes from within

Chapter 2

How Are You?

How many times do you hear this and respond 'I'm fine'? What would you really like to say?

Begin your journal with the honest answer to this question. Take as long as you need. These are your private pages; a place where you can be completely honest. It may take five minutes, half an hour or an hour every day for the next week or month. Do this now. The next stage will mean so much more when your thoughts and feelings are on the pages in front of you.

> **Begin your journal**
>
> ➔ write about your health
>
> ➔ write about your feelings
>
> ➔ write about how you see your life now

Now complete the following, creating a snapshot of how you feel about your life right now.

> **Complete the following**
>
> Circle the number that reflects how much you feel in control of your life. (Where 1 = not at all in control and 10 = completely in control)
>
> 1   2   3   4   5   6   7   8   9   10
>
> Circle the number that reflects how much choice you feel you have in your life. (Where 1 = no choice at all, and 10 = I have complete choice in everything I do)
>
> 1   2   3   4   5   6   7   8   9   10
>
> Circle the number that reflects your sense of opportunity in life. (Where 1 = I see no new opportunities for my life, and 10 = my life is filled with new opportunities)
>
> 1   2   3   4   5   6   7   8   9   10

'How are you?' is the first question I ask when I start this course with a group. The people are different each time, and the symptoms they experience very individual, but I know they'll be feeling:

- frustrated, angry, depressed, guilty
- an enormous sense of loss
- pessimistic about the future

How do I know this? Because these feelings are common to most people with M.E. or Chronic Fatigue Syndrome. Let's explore yours some more.

Read pages 1 and 2 of your journal

What stands out...

- negative feelings such as frustration, anger, depression, guilt?

    - mark each one with a coloured highlighter

- or positive feelings such as hope, fulfilment, contentment?

    - mark each one with a different highlighter

Look at those pages – which colour stands out?

- the one highlighting how negative life is?
- or the one highlighting how positive life is?

If it's mainly positive, that's great. You're already well on the way to providing the best possible healing environment for your body.

If it's mainly negative, that's great. You're already well on the way to providing the best possible healing environment for your body.

This isn't a printing error!

Wherever you are right now is the best possible starting point for you. Even depression, maybe most of all depression, is a perfect springboard for change. More on this later.

You are not your illness.

This course is about rediscovering the real 'you'. Just now you may be feeling overwhelmed by the thoughts and feelings that go hand-in-hand with illness. Begin the first exercise and all those negative thoughts and feelings, that have been consuming your energy, will be flowing onto those pages - not trapped inside you. Take a look at those thoughts and feelings:

- see them as separate from you
- see them as a normal reaction to a physically and emotionally challenging time

Sleepless nights with the same thoughts going round and round in your mind and the black days when you can't see how it's ever going to change, are a perfectly normal reaction to an unwanted disruption to your life. It would be strange if you weren't feeling as you do.

This understandable reaction is a great starting point.

As uncomfortable as they are, these thoughts and feelings have kick-started a very important journey for you - your road to recovery.

Now the question becomes - what next?

You've probably tried different therapies. Whether or not they help doesn't just depend on how often you go or the skill of the therapist. Take a look at these examples, adding your own experiences.

- you join a yoga class but start to miss sessions
- your plan to rest every day after lunch somehow gets lost before the end of the week
- you never quite get round to talking with your boss about reducing your hours

You may not be aware of it, but these situations, and probably many others, are the result of unconscious choices you are making.

All sorts of things will be influencing those choices. Exploring these influences is fundamental to this course.

There's a proven relationship between stress and illness.

The close link between mind and body means that the way you think about things can bring about physical changes. Replay a stressful event in your mind. Do it, now. Pitch yourself into a situation where you felt really uncomfortable. How did your body react? Did your heart start racing? Was your stomach churning? Did you get a dry mouth? Did you tense up?

What's happening?

- when you feel threatened, your body triggers the short term 'fight or flight' stress response through a combination of nerve and hormonal signals involving the hypothalamus, pituitary and adrenal glands

- long term activation of this stress response can disrupt many of the body's processes, including the immune, digestive, nervous and cardio-vascular systems

- when immune system dysfunction persists, the body may become locked into a downward spiral, leaving you susceptible to ongoing illness

Consider this comment by William Leith.[1]

'... it's not germs that make us ill. Rather, when we become ill, germs come and get us. Then, as we know, doctors try to get rid of the germs. But maybe they would be doing a better job if they examined the conditions that enabled the germs to thrive.'

What does this mean?

When illness strikes, it's likely that your immune system has already been weakened by environmental, physical, emotional or mental stress. Any kind of stress:

- actively undermines your immune system
- disrupts your body's efforts to restore itself to health
- interferes with your ability to benefit from treatment
- is a major energy drain

An awareness of the triggers that create stress in you, and your personal reaction to those triggers, is a vital first step in recovering your health.

---

[1] Writing in the Daily Telegraph.

> **What causes you to feel stressed?**
>
> When you feel stressed, ask yourself:
>
> - what is causing the stress?
> - what thoughts are going through my mind?
> - how do I feel, physically and emotionally

When an illness becomes chronic, it's natural to focus on your symptoms and become anxious about what's causing them and why your body feels as it does. This is stressful.

You probably compare your symptoms with those of fellow sufferers, trying to make sense of the changes that have taken place. You look to your GP or therapists for treatments that will work. But, more often than not, these experts are as mystified as you about how to treat this illness.

Constant questioning and looking for answers outside of yourself can lead to a build-up of frustration, anger and depression. The immune system is further weakened by the stress caused by these emotions and a vicious cycle begins.

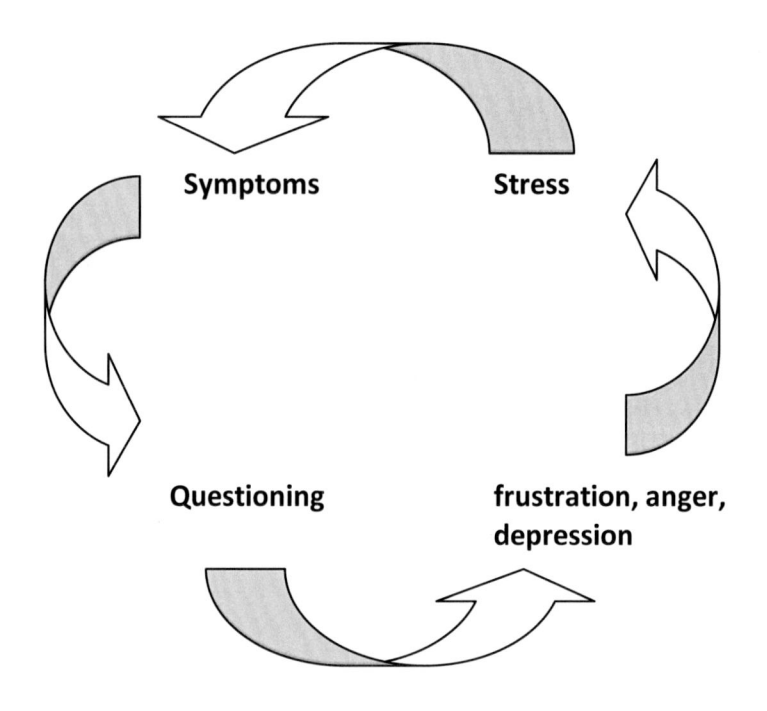

```
        Symptoms  →  Stress
           ↑            ↓
       Questioning ← frustration, anger,
                      depression
```

Which brings you to your first choice:

- to remain locked in this cycle
  or
- to focus on constantly releasing stress and tension to free up valuable energy for healing

This second option is positive, effective action *you* can take *right now* to make a difference to your life.

Begin with a technique that's unbelievably easy, free and

takes hardly any time. It's a most effective way to relieve stress.

Read through the following[2] several times, find a private and comfortable spot, close your eyes and complete the exercise. It's easy to remember and only takes five minutes.

> **Take Five**
>
> Close your eyes
>
> S M I L E - broadly
>
> In a moment, take 3 deep breaths
> As you breathe in, say to yourself – release
> As you breathe out, say to yourself – and relax
>
> Then continue breathing normally
>
> Now focus on your scalp and think – relax
> focus on your face – let your cheek muscles relax
> focus on your jaw – let your mouth open slightly
> focus on your shoulders – let them drop
> focus on your abdomen – relax your stomach
> focus on your bottom – unclench those muscles

---

[2] Inspired by the work of Louise Hay, Patricia Crane and others

focus on your arms and hands – let them feel heavy
focus on your legs and feet – let them feel heavy

Feel a wave of relaxation sweep from head to toe

Know that you are in the right place at the right time doing exactly the right thing

Things are as they are
Life is as it is
For now

Just for the moment, give your body permission to be exactly as it is
Just for the moment, give yourself permission to feel exactly as you feel

Your body and mind are doing their very best with how things are right now

You are doing your very best with how things are right now

S M I L E

Take one more deep breath and open your eyes

'Take Five' as often as possible during the day.

Other invaluable techniques for releasing stress include:

- deep breathing
- relaxation
- meditation
- yoga
- Tai Chi
- avoiding stimulants
- avoiding pressurised situations
- pacing yourself

I recommend making deep breathing and relaxation part of your daily routine. Why? Because these simple techniques encourage your body to:

- switch off your sympathetic nervous system, which produces the stress response of muscle tension, increased heart rate, shallow breathing, increased blood pressure, racing mind

- and engage the parasympathetic nervous system, which produces the relaxation response where muscles relax, breathing deepens, brain waves change

Deep breathing.

When you experience the stress response your breathing

becomes shallow. Expanding your lungs increases the flow of much needed oxygen, bringing more energy into your system. This is something *you* can do *right now* to reduce your daily response to stress and improve your health and well-being.

> **Practise deep breathing**
>
> At regular intervals throughout the day, and immediately when you are feeling stressed, practise deep breathing. To know if you are doing this effectively:
>
> ➜ place one hand on your chest and the other just above your belly button
>
> ➜ breathe in
>
> ➜ observe which hand moves the most
>
> ➜ deepen your breathing until your lower hand is moving more than your top hand
>
> ➜ Take six deep breaths and then allow your breathing to relax into its natural pattern
>
> ➜ Repeat several times a day

Relaxation.

This is another effective technique for reducing stress. Create a comfortable, undisturbed space for yourself and put on one of the many CDs available that will guide you through around twenty minutes of deep relaxation. It may take practise to quieten your mind, but make this an essential part of your daily routine and it will happen.[3]

It's easy to put off doing something new. Decide now when you will buy or download the CD. Once you have it, put reminders to listen wherever you'll see them. Place them together with a picture of something you'll do when you're feeling a bit better.

Regularly practise deep breathing and relaxation and you will:
- reduce your stress levels
- prevent further stress building up
- make more energy available for healing

Now is a good time to take a break. Why? Because:

- mental activity is as exhausting as physical activity
- it's important to pace yourself

During this break, 'Take Time' for yourself.

'Taking Time' is an essential part of this course. A major obstacle to recovery is an unconscious inability to make

---

[3] For example, 'Reducing Stress is an Inside Job' by Patricia Crane

self-care a priority. This simple technique ensures your health and well-being receives the attention it needs.

What is 'Taking Time'? Very simply, it's putting aside a block of time, an hour, an afternoon or an entire day, to do something by yourself. It's taking time out from obligations, responsibilities or the expectations of others; time that is purely and exclusively yours.

This may be a new experience for you. Maybe you're accustomed to putting others first, missing out on nurturing yourself.

You are not your illness. You are a unique individual with hopes and dreams to fulfil. But illness may have caused you to lose sight of that individual. 'Taking Time' will help you to restore balance by re-focusing on yourself.

Resist the temptation to choose something you used to love doing but know you can't do now. This will only reinforce your sense of loss. However overwhelming the illness feels, there is something you can do for yourself. If you had no-one else to consider what would you do? If it's something completely new that's even better.

For 'Taking Time' to be effective it's vital that anything you choose isn't a:
- should
- ought
- have to
- or must

And is:
- fun
- easily within reach
- and a treat

Decide on an hour, an afternoon or a day, the more the better, and ring-fence that time. Block it out in your diary so others can see it is taken.

This time is non-negotiable. You have a commitment that cannot be broken. That commitment is to yourself, or to put it another way, to your Self.

A few ideas:

- go for a ride on the top of a bus
- go to the pictures in the middle of the day
- have morning coffee in the best hotel in town
- day dream
- buy modelling clay and try some self-expression
- try painting by numbers
- create a mosaic
- visit an art gallery
- have a bubble bath
- take a camera and capture some portraits
- write a poem
- have a massage
- play a game

This is YOUR time - Enjoy - You deserve it!

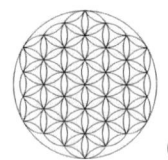

CHAPTER 2 SUMMARY

- Negative thoughts and feelings are great for helping you to become aware of your needs
- Where you are right now is the perfect starting point
- There's a proven relationship between stress and illness
- Constantly releasing stress and tension will free up valuable energy for healing
- 'Taking Time' is fundamental to this course

ACTIONS

- Highlight the negatives and positives in your writing
- Identify what causes you to feel stressed
- Practise 'Take 5', deep breathing and relaxation at every opportunity
- 'Take Time' for yourself

Chapter 3

Forecasting Your Day

What is Stress?

In the last chapter we looked at how you can release stress and tension. But what exactly is stress?

Imagine yourself in a situation many find stressful. You're stuck in a traffic jam on a motorway on your way to a vital business or family event. You can't see what's caused it and have no alternative but to sit and wait. What are you thinking?

- just my luck
- my boss/partner/family will be furious
- I'm letting them down

How are you feeling?

- tense, willing something to move?
- angry at life, fate, the cars in front?
- upset at letting others down

Maybe your mind is telling you that of course you feel angry, anxious, upset. Anyone would be when their day had been ruined, their job put on the line or their relationship undermined. Of course you feel stressed!

This may be what your mind is telling you but you have a choice about whether or not to believe it. There's another, more positive way of thinking that will reduce stress and conserve energy.

There are actually two parts to this situation. And your thoughts are the key to unravelling them. Consider this:

Part 1: That you are stuck in a traffic jam is a *fact* that *cannot* be changed.

Part 2: That you feel stressed is the result of a *thought* that *you can* change.

As Epictetus, a Greek philosopher, put it: *Men are disturbed not by things that happen, but by their opinions of the things that happen*.

We all have a verbal tape playing in our minds. Every second of every day (and night!) the voice on this tape provides a commentary on your life. Your thoughts create this commentary, transforming what is *actually* happening into your *experience* of what is happening.

> ## Become aware of your personal tape
>
> - think of something you do several times a day like preparing food, using the computer, etc.
>
> - each time you perform this action, pause
>
> - what are you thinking?
>
> - are your thoughts positive or negative?

For example, as you stand to prepare some food you might realise that you're thinking:

- *why can't I even cook a meal without feeling exhausted?*
- *I can't do anything*
- *What's the point?*

STOP
Are these thoughts negative or positive?

Being caught up with negative thoughts is very common with M.E. or Chronic Fatigue Syndrome and is a massive energy drain, undermining your body's ability to heal.

This is how it works:

> Thoughts of anger or resentment stimulate
> the stress response which,
> in the absence of any real danger...

> becomes a major stress on your body

> and an overwhelming energy drain

If feeling stressed is a constant factor in your life then what little resources you do have are being depleted, unconsciously undermining your body's attempts to heal.

It doesn't have to be this way. Remember, it's not what's happening that's creating stress... but your thoughts about what's happening.

The facts are clear - you're having difficulty preparing a meal. But your thoughts and emotions are something else; they are a reaction to the facts, interpreting them as something to worry or get angry about.

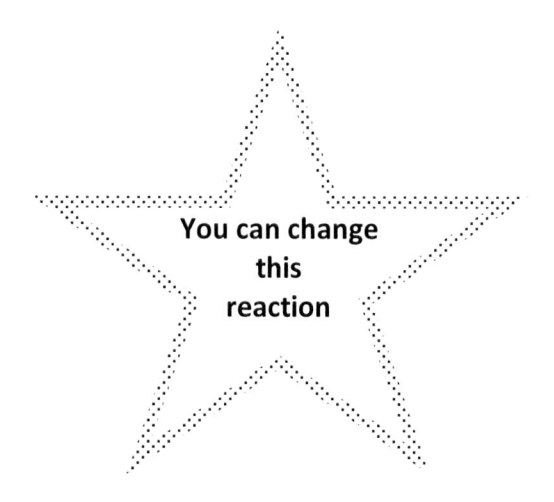

You can change this reaction

How?
By following 4 simple steps. As soon as you feel the slightest stress:

Step 1 take immediate action to diffuse your stress reaction -'Take Five', breathe deeply, relax.
Step 2 become aware of the negative thoughts that caused this reaction.
Step 3 realise that you can replace these with more positive thoughts.
Step 4 and do it!

Changing negative thoughts into positive thoughts.

As you listen to the tape playing in your mind, you'll become more and more aware of when you're locked into negative thoughts. By realising you're becoming stressed and doing something about it you stop the stress reaction in its tracks.
But what then? How do you actually change negative thoughts for more positive ones? Some weather forecasting will help.

What is *actually* happening?

- you look out the window and see it's raining - that's what is *actually* happening

- but your internal tape, your thought, may be saying, 'Oh, no, not another miserable day'

- how does that negative thought make you feel? Miserable?

Your thought is influencing how you *experience* what's happening, that is, how you feel.

It isn't a miserable day, it's simply raining. Your feelings have been determined by your thoughts, by the tape running through your mind, not by the weather outside your window.

But your internal tape has been running for so long you don't question it any more. You believe it's a miserable day.

The good news is – you can change the tape.

And as your thoughts change, so too will your feelings. This practical way of releasing negative thoughts and feelings will free up much needed energy to help your recovery and is something *you* can do *right now* to make a difference to your life.

Forecasting your day

Weather forecasters use neutral words because another week without rain may be great for the tourist industry but a disaster for farmers.

- first thing every morning, describe the weather as it actually is

- make your words a description, not a judgement

- instead of *'what a miserable day,'* try, *'it's overcast today'*

After a week or two of weather forecasting you'll become aware of a subtle change in your thinking. Looking through the window at a damp, misty day your first response might be, *'it's misty today'* instead of, *'oh no, not another depressing day'*.

- *'Oh, no, not another depressing day,'* is a powerfully negative thought that's bound to leave you feeling miserable or worse
- *'It's misty today,'* is a neutral thought that will leave you feeling relatively okay

Let's return to our example of preparing food. As you stand with a pile of half-peeled potatoes in front of you and your mind starts to play its negative tape – PAUSE. Become aware of any stress these negative thoughts are creating in your body and follow **The Four Steps:**

Step 1 'Take Five', breathe and relax.
Step 2 Identify the negative thought that created the stress response: *'I can't do anything'*.
Step 3 Remember – you can change this thought.
Step 4 And do it, opting for a more neutral, less judgemental thought: *'It's not true that I can't do anything. I simply need to sit down for a moment'*.

Try the same process with our traffic jam example.

Step 1 'Take Five', breathe and relax.
Step 2 Identify the negative thoughts that created the

stress response: *'I should have known the traffic would be bad. Trust me to screw up – again!'*

Step 3 Remember - you can change these thoughts.

Step 4 And do it, opting for a neutral, less judgemental thought: *'There's been a build up of traffic that means I can't move for the moment. It's perfectly understandable that I'll be arriving later than expected'.*

Remember:

Part 1 That you are in a traffic jam is a description of your current circumstances, a simple fact.

Part 2 That traffic jams are stressful is a judgement you've unconsciously chosen to link to this situation.

The stress has been created by your thoughts, by the tape running through your mind, not by the traffic jam.

Creating daylight between an internal tape, that's so familiar you're probably no longer aware of it, and the facts, gives you a powerful tool for change. After a lifetime of reacting automatically to events, suddenly you have a choice every time you feel stressed.

Option 1 To succumb to powerfully negative thoughts that leave you feeling tense, angry, anxious or exhausted.

Option 2 To opt for positive, nurturing thoughts that leave you feeling relatively calm, optimistic and energised.

Force of habit is so strong it may not feel as though you have a choice. But you do! Try it. Next time you're stuck in a traffic jam and start to feel stressed:

- think 'STOP: there's another way I can look at this'
- think – Four steps

Imagine you're the person waiting. You might have your own reasons for being irritated or disappointed but you wouldn't be justified in blaming the person sitting in the car.

So do what you can - 'phone to say you'll be late - then let yourself off the hook. Instead of getting carried away with negative thoughts such as, *'what will they think of me'* or *'I've messed up again'*, which can be strangely satisfying, focus on the positives. You've time to take a drink, chat, notice the scenery, close your eyes, relax, enjoy having nothing to do.

Out of sight the jam will be freeing up and when you do move on you'll be relaxed and energised instead of wrung out with tension and anxiety.

Remember

when you become aware of your thoughts

⬇

you can begin to change those thoughts

⬇

which changes your experience of situations

⬇

which reduces stress

⬇

which supports recovery

Illness can be like a traffic jam.

Your circumstances are as they are - for the moment. But, although it may not feel like it, you do have a choice about how to respond to those circumstances. And up ahead, just out of sight, things are freeing up.

We'll explore this more later in the course but for now, simply become aware that every second of every day you're making choices, often automatically and unconsciously; choices that sometimes undermine rather than support your recovery.

By following the exercises in this course you're becoming aware of those choices and discovering how to change them.

And speaking of choices... did you 'Take Time' for yourself?

- what did you do, how long did it take, how did you feel?

- if you didn't take time for yourself, why not?

- did you forget, either to do it or what it was you'd decided to do?

- did other things eat into the time you'd set aside for yourself?

Write your answers in your journal.

Decide how you will 'Take Time' for yourself now.

You may want to repeat your last choice, or do something completely different. Whatever you choose, remember this is *your* time. So during the next hour, this afternoon or one day this week, take time to do something that is:

- fun
- easily within your reach
- and a treat

Make sure that no:

- should's
- ought's
- have to's
- or must's

...creep in anywhere. Yes, the cupboard under the stairs might need clearing out and I'm sure you'll feel a lot better when it's done, but that's another action plan for another day.

This time is to feed the inner 'you' that's always wanted to try archery or visit a National Trust property. And make sure this is *your* time. No gate crashers. This is not a time for compromising to keep others happy. The only consideration is what *you* want to do.

End of story.
Enjoy!

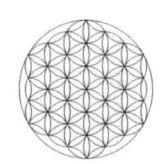

CHAPTER 3 SUMMARY

➔ Becoming aware of your personal reaction to stress is a vital first step

➔ Illness can be like a traffic jam - your circumstances are as they are, for the moment at least - but you can choose how you respond to them

➔ Choose to replace thoughts that leave you feeling tense, anxious or frustrated with thoughts that help you to remain calm, peaceful, relaxed

ACTIONS

➔ Every morning, describe the weather as it actually is

➔ Explore your personal stress reaction

➔ Become aware of your personal tape

➔ Practise 'Taking Time'

Chapter 4

The Power of Choice

Why is this course so important for you?

You are a unique expression of life. No-one sees life through your eyes or has the unique combination of personality and experience that you have. Your life is too precious to be lived in the shadows.

Charles Handy once said: *'What other life have I yet to discover?'* As you read this text and practise the exercises, you'll discover a new sense of optimism about your life and the possibilities that lie ahead.

How are you getting on?

When you feel stressed, I asked you to explore:

- the exact circumstances
- the thoughts going through your mind
- how you feel, physically and emotionally

What have you discovered about the thoughts that go through your mind when you're stressed? How do these thoughts make you feel? Anxious? Tense? Exhausted? Do you want to continue to feel this way? Or do you want to start right now to reduce stress and the toll it takes on your body?

Because you've reacted to stress in the same way for so long it will feel like an automatic process, like a domino run that, once started, seems unstoppable. But now you have a way of removing the crucial tile that will stop that domino run in its tracks; The Four Steps. Use them all the time to change your reaction to stress, including any caused by the illness itself.

Step 1 'Take Five', breathe and relax.
Step 2 Identify the negative thoughts causing the stress. *'I'm never going to get my life back. What's the point?'*
Step 3 Remember, you can change these thoughts – they're a real pain anyway!
Step 4 And do it. Think positive. *'I'll follow this course and do everything I can to support my recovery.'*

Practising these steps will help you become more aware of when you've been taken over by your old stress reaction... and how easy it is to change it! And the more you do it, the easier it becomes. Decide right now that when you feel stressed you'll:

- pause
- and follow The Four Steps

I know this course can make a difference to your life. But whether or not it does is a matter of *choice*. Your choice.

You may be finding that:

- you know it's a good idea to reduce stress
- you have the information to do it
- and you'd like to do it
- but somehow it doesn't happen

Why not?

All action, or inaction, is the result of choices you are making at some level.

Every second of every day you're making choices, usually unconsciously. Sometimes these choices undermine rather than support your recovery. Why might this be happening?

The Power of Automatic Pilot.

Consider this. You need to drive to town for an urgent appointment. Just before you leave you remind yourself that road works are causing delays on the most direct route so it would be sensible to go another way. Yet a few minutes later you're stuck in a queue at the temporary traffic lights cursing yourself for forgetting to take a different route.

Why? What affected your ability to make the best choice despite having all the facts?

The Force of Habit.

The force of habit is created through constantly doing things the same way. It's difficult to resist. In the above example, you probably switched to automatic pilot as soon as you got into the car. Any new information was simply no match for the force of habit. You did what you always do.

Habit is your default setting, the unconscious way you'll think and behave unless you consciously make a different choice. This takes practice.

If you allow habit or unconscious patterns - that is the way you always drive to town - to continue despite a change in circumstances - road works taking place - you'll come unstuck - an increase in stress levels because you're late.

How does this apply to M.E. or Chronic Fatigue Syndrome?

If you allow an unconscious pattern - for example, overworking - to continue despite a change in circumstances - your body and mind not responding as before - then you'll come unstuck - continuing or worsening symptoms.

> **Becoming Aware (1)**
>
> As you go through the day, reflect on the decisions (choices) you are making. Do they:
>
> - reduce tension and stress, supporting your body's healing
>
>   **or**
> - create stress and tension, undermining your body's healing?

For example.

Are you great at meeting other people's needs but not so good at meeting your own? Maybe you're unconsciously making choices that create stress by:

- not eating well, resting enough, exercising appropriately
- not taking enough 'time out' from responsibilities
- not having enough fun
- not seeking emotional support to help you through difficult times
- not looking after yourself when there's a lot on at work or at home

You need rest and relaxation, emotional and physical

expression, meaning and purpose in your life. If you neglect any of these your body may react by getting or remaining ill.

IMPORTANT.

If you discover that, due to force of habit, you're not making the best choices for yourself, **do not use this information to beat yourself up**. You're doing the very best you can with the awareness that you have. And as your awareness grows you will choose to do things differently.

The most important choice you can make is to pay attention to yourself, or to put it another way, to your Self. Right now, there is nothing more important than your health and well-being.

You are a unique, wonderful expression of life. Anything that interferes with your ability to express yourself, such as M.E. or Chronic Fatigue Syndrome, is a sign that it's time to respond to your Self as never before.

You are not your illness or your reactions to it. You're a person with hopes, dreams and a life to live. You may have lost sight of that person but you're there - waiting to be rediscovered.

Are you willing to put yourself first?

The voice on your internal tape may be saying:

- *that's so selfish!*
- *who am I to deserve special treatment?*
- *how can I with children around or work to complete?*

These sound-bites have probably been around for a long time, making themselves heard whenever you're tempted to put your own needs first. They're so familiar you don't question them anymore.

But just because they're familiar doesn't mean they're right.

As we grow up we adopt beliefs from those around us by listening to the things they say and watching the things they do. We might rebel later on but only after years of believing that if the all powerful adults in our lives say and do these things they must be right. Mustn't they?

But what if your parents only believed it was selfish to put themselves first because that's what their parents believed, and so on back through the generations?

Because beliefs get stuck in a family tree it doesn't mean they're right for you.

Sometimes it goes beyond beliefs to judgements made about us that we take to heart. Any of these sound familiar?

- *leave that alone, you'll only make a mess of it*
- *whatever made you think you could........?*
- *I want doesn't get*

Before long we start believing what we're told. And even worse, we make a recording of the original and replay it over and over way into adulthood! Maybe it's always there, reminding you time and time again that everyone else is more important or more capable than you.

Putting others first is a great choice to make… when it's not at the expense of your own needs and is truly your choice.

Take a fresh look at the beliefs being replayed on your tape and ask, 'which are preventing me from putting myself first, from making my recovery my top priority'.

Becoming Aware (2)

The next time a negative sound-bite plays on your internal tape, stop and ask:

- do I really believe this?

- is this belief stopping me from responding to my needs or expressing myself?

Michelangelo is credited with saying:

> *Creating the David was easy. All I had to do was chip away all that was not David from the stone.*

Rediscovering your energy goes hand in hand with rediscovering your Self; chipping away everything you've picked up along the way that's obscuring the real you.

What's the voice on your tape saying right now?

The negative voice may be so familiar you'll experience a lot of resistance to letting it go. The tape will keep rewinding to make sure you're still buying into it. Maybe it's saying:

- *that's rubbish, it's this illness that's making my life a misery*
- *I'm not imagining this! My life is filled with pain*
- *this illness has robbed me of everything I loved*

How do you separate yourself from this negative voice?

By using the Power of Choice:

Choice 1: You allow negative thoughts and feelings to feed your belief that life is awful and you're powerless to change it.

Choice 2: You recognise that your negative internal tape is creating a miserable experience of life... and resolve to change it.

Practise 'Taking Time'

Practise putting yourself first by choosing to do something:

- ➔ you enjoy
- ➔ is easily within your reach
- ➔ and a treat

Take another look at the list in Chapter 3 for ideas or create your own.

It's your choice.

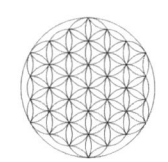

CHAPTER 4 SUMMARY

- What other life have you yet to discover?
- Use The Four Steps to reduce stress
- All action - or inaction - reflects choices you're making at a conscious or unconscious level
- Force of habit affects your ability to make the best choices
- Choose to put yourself first
- Rediscovering your energy goes hand in hand with rediscovering your Self

ACTIONS

- Practise becoming aware of, and changing, your internal tape
- Develop a new awareness
- Choose to 'Take Time' in a thoroughly enjoyable way

Chapter 5

Boom and Bust

Are you 'Taking Time'?

What did you do? How did you feel? Did you forget? Some common responses in the groups are:

- I really enjoyed having permission to do what I wanted
- I didn't get round to it. I don't know why
- we had visitors and when they'd gone I didn't have the energy
- I did it but felt guilty taking time away from the family
- it felt so selfish, but wonderful!
- I just had too much on at work to take the time
- how can I do something for me when it takes two hours just to get dressed?

In the last chapter I said all action, or inaction, is a reflection of choices you make at a conscious or unconscious level. Are you choosing to 'Take Time'?

If *yes*... congratulations!
If *no*... what's stopping you?

- is it because you had visitors... or were you unable to say that you were taking some time for yourself?

- is it that work is too busy... or did you place this activity at the bottom of your list of priorities?

Most of the time it won't feel like a choice. It will feel as though circumstances are making those choices for you – the visitors, the workload, etc.

There is another way of looking at this.

Take the situation of visitors arriving for the weekend. If you were alone you'd be resting by midday. But entertaining visitors probably means preparing lunch then taking them into town, to the park or a local National Trust house; all the while concentrating, talking and even more draining, listening.

What do you do? My guess is that you often push beyond the point where you know you should stop, knowing you'll pay for it later. The more this happens, the more you become locked into a pattern of boom and bust and the more entrenched the illness becomes.

How do you change this pattern?

Step 1 Keep a record of *when, where* and *how* you're spending your energy now.

I recommend the daily diary described by Dr. Darrell Ho Yen[4]. Using a banking analogy of credit and expenditure, you'll see exactly where you're 'overspending'.

Take two pages in your journal for each day. On the left hand side, at the beginning of each day, assess how much energy you think you have to spend; how much you feel able to do. This is your credit. On the right hand side, at the end of the day, write two or three lines about how you've spent your energy. This is your expenditure.

On the credit side give yourself a score of between 1 and 10 where 1 = expecting to have severe symptoms at rest, in bed all day, feeling unable to do anything and 10 = expecting to feel completely well and lead a normal life. This score is not about what you *can* do, simply what you *think* you can do.

On the expenditure side be as precise and factual as you can. For example, some of my early entries were:

Sat 25th	3	Gardening 1hr. Reading 2hr. Bath. Evening concert. 2hrs. Sludgy day
Sun 26th	3	Bad night. Awake every 2 hrs. 30mins reading. 1hr listening to radio. Cooking & eating lunch. 1.5hrs, visitors. Driving & shopping, 2hrs. TV 1hr. Exhausted all day.

---
[4] Better Recovery from Viral Illness. Dr Darrell Ho Yen

Mon 27th	4	Car trip to Plymouth. 2hrs at Auction. Stayed up with visitors. Shattered.
Tues 28th	3	Broken night. Computer 1.5hrs Reading 1hr. Prepared lunch. Reading 1hr. TV 2hrs. Long phone call. Shattered.
Wed 29th	4	College by 9.30. 6hrs concentrating, talking, driving there & back. Prepared tea. Straight to bed. Desperate, so exhausted.
Thurs 30th	4	Morning studying. Prepared lunch. Completely wasted rest of the day.
Fri 31st	3	Reading 30mins. Shower. Town 1hr. Prepared lunch 2hrs talking to visitors. Prepared tea. Zombie After.

The 3's and 4's were my estimate of how much energy I thought I had to spend each day. How wrong was I! My 'end of the day' comments said it all. Shattered. Exhausted. Zombie.

More than twelve weeks into the diary I wrote: *I'm not surprised I'm still ill, look at everything I'm doing. I'm not giving myself complete and utter down time to heal. I can't blame anyone else if I'm exhausted. LEARN THE LESSON!*

It took this daily diary to make me realise I was constantly 'overspending'.

Step 2 Look at your activity record and, thinking of the left column as credit and the right as expenditure, ask yourself each day:

- have I overspent?
- am I living on overdraft?

Living on overdraft is not sustainable. If you keep making choices that leave you overspent at the end of every day you are undermining your body's attempts to heal.

Never spend 110% of your energy. Only ever 80%. What you save today will re-charge your batteries and make more energy available further down the line. Use the information in your diary to do this. For example, I decided not to do long stints on the computer until I was scoring 4's every day. I also wrote at the top of my pages:

STOP before the battery begins to dim.
Do not drive on to the end of the task.

My initial scores were all 3/4. A few months later they were 6/7 and I was adjusting my activity as I went, most of the time! Listing everything that demanded energy - cooking, talking on the phone, working on the computer, listening - made me much more conscious of where I could save.

Crucially, I waited until the right hand column told me I felt fine at the end of the day before I increased my activity.

> **Start Banking**
>
> - make a commitment to keep a diary
> - each day ask 'Am I over-spending?'
> - identify when you need to stop to stay within your energy credit
> - as soon as you get the slightest inkling of the battery dimming... STOP
>   - avoid the 'I'll just finish this' syndrome

If the sentence, '*I'll just finish this…*' crosses your mind, your body is already whispering, '*please stop*'.

Do not over-ride that plea.

If you do, your body will need to shout louder next time and you may find yourself forced out of action for days instead of choosing to rest for a short while.

Are you thinking, '*easier said than done*'? Why might you push beyond the point where your body is telling you to stop? We've already looked at how habit overrides your conscious choices – remember the road works? Other responses in the groups include:

- *I'm fed up with being a kill-joy all the time*
- *why shouldn't I enjoy myself?*
- *they expect me to entertain them*
- *they get fed up with me saying no all the time*
- *I feel so out of it if I rest*
- *I don't get much pleasure; it's worth the price*

These may sound familiar; they may not. Either way, a crucial step in freeing yourself from this damaging pattern of boom and bust is to discover why you push beyond the point when your body is telling you to stop.

But first, remind yourself of the 'Take Five' exercise.

Take Five

Close your eyes.
S M I L E - broadly.

In a moment, take 3 deep breaths
As you breathe in, say to yourself – release
As you breathe out, say to yourself – and relax

Continue breathing normally

focus on your scalp and think – relax
focus on your face – relax your cheek muscles
focus on your jaw – relax so your mouth opens
focus on your shoulders – let them drop

focus on your abdomen – relax your stomach
focus on your bottom – unclench those muscles
focus on your arms and hands – let them flop and feel heavy
focus on your legs and feet – let them flop and feel heavy

Feel a wave of relaxation sweep your body

Know that you are in the right place at the right time doing exactly the right thing
Things are as they are
Life is as it is
For now

Just for the moment, give your body permission to be exactly as it is
Just for the moment, give yourself permission to feel exactly as you feel

Your body and mind are doing their very best with how things are right now

You are doing your very best with how things are right now

S M I L E

Take a deep breath and open your eyes

'Take Five' as often as you can during the day. Do it when you wake, after breakfast, every time you have a cup of tea, when you go to bed, every time you feel tense, angry, miserable or exhausted. It's impossible to do this too much. It frees up energy for healing and is a great technique for relaxing body and mind sufficiently to expand your self-awareness.

Self-awareness is about discovering:

- why you do what you do
- why you don't do what you don't do

There's a great saying that goes, *'if you always do what you always did, you'll always get what you always got'*.

- does pushing yourself too hard work?
- do you feel better for longer as a result?
- is it logical to continue doing this?

When I ask these questions in a group the unanimous answer is - **NO!** Which leads us to the next question. Why squander the energy you do have instead of using it to underpin your recovery? Consider the following:

Thought: *I push myself because I want to feel normal again.*
Response: It's great that you want to feel well, and do you?
For a while, yes.

And how will you feel tomorrow?
Exhausted, drained, really down.
What matters most? Feeling well today and not tomorrow or feeling well all the time?
Feeling well all the time.
So why do you choose to just feel well today?
Because something is better than nothing.
Are you aware of the banking theory? Never spend 110% of your energy. Only ever 80%. What you save today will re-charge your batteries and make more available for longer a little further down the line.
Yes.
Do you believe this?
Yes.
But your actions say you don't.
I suppose not.
What stops you acting on this good advice? What is driving you to squander the energy you do have? Search for a feeling.
Maybe I'm afraid I'll never be well. I have to keep proving to myself that I'm not really ill. That I can be okay, if only for an hour.
So you make choices you know will make you worse because you're afraid you'll never get better. **Your choices are being driven by fear, not by love and care for yourself**.

Maybe this sequence reflects your thoughts, maybe it doesn't. Explore the unconscious choices you are making.

> **Recall the last time you overdid it**
>
> Think about the exact circumstances:
>
> ➡ where were you?
>
> ➡ what had just happened?
>
> ➡ what thoughts were going through your mind?

Write about this situation in your journal in as much detail as you can, read it back and then answer these questions:

➡ what unconscious choice do you now realise you made?

➡ why did you make that choice?

Repeat this process each time you overdo it and suffer the consequences. Develop the habit of taking out your journal and writing about each incident in detail. Then look at your writing. Really look. Beyond the words, beyond your immediate thoughts, look for the unconscious choices you're making. What are they and why might you be making them?

For example, perhaps you discover you overdo things because you simply can't leave a job unfinished.

Let this insight lead to a question:

- Q. Why can't I leave a job unfinished?
- A. It irritates me to see things unfinished
- Q. Why?
- A. I like to do things right
- Q. Why?
- A. I don't know, I just do!

Don't worry if you get stuck. Maybe it's an echo of a powerful adult instilling the belief in you that if you start something you must finish it. We'll explore some possibilities further on.

Meanwhile, simply practise raising your awareness step by step.

Raise your awareness

Every time you over-ride messages from your body:

→ catch the thoughts going through your mind

→ write these down in your journal

Don't put yourself under any pressure to change your reactions, it will soon become second nature to respond differently. For now, you're an observer, collecting data on the unconscious thoughts and feelings that have led to choices that undermine your body's attempts to heal.

Read the last paragraph again.

In the first sentence I talk about your *reactions* then your *response*. One of the best ways to use your new awareness is to practise changing a **negative reaction** into a **positive response.**

When you run out of energy:

- ➜ a *reaction* would be to become angry that this illness has stopped you doing what you want to do... again!

- ➜ a *response* would be to become aware that your body needs to rest, and to make a positive choice to do that

Like the rain, tiredness isn't maliciously depriving you of anything, it's simply a message to rest and reflect.

What thoughts are playing on your internal tape right now? Maybe:

- ➜ *...but I don't want to rest, I want to live*
- ➜ *I want to work, to be involved in sport, to socialise*
- ➜ *I don't want to be limited by my body like this*

What emotions are these thoughts creating? Anger? Frustration? Despair? All of the above! Your internal tape may constantly remind you of everything you could do before you were ill that you can't do now and how miserable that makes you feel.

These feelings are common to many suffering from M.E. or Chronic Fatigue Syndrome ... and are one of the biggest obstacles to recovery.

They drain you of energy, perpetuate resistance, which is no more than fighting your own body, and lock you into a pattern of boom and bust.

Through this course you're discovering how to change that negative reaction into a positive response, rediscovering harmony with your body and working with it to create a life worth living.

Go back over the essential exercises. Give them another try and see old unwanted habits begin to lose their grip.

And finally.

Take some time out from all the reading and reflection and give yourself permission to enjoy 'Taking Time' ensuring it is fun, easily within your reach and a treat

A few more ideas:

- lie on the sofa or the grass and look for shapes in the clouds
- buy a calligraphy kit
- go for a paddle
- rediscover jigsaws
- kick up some autumn leaves
- write a children's story
- take close-ups of textured tree barks or flower petals
- sing along to your favourite tracks... really loudly!

It's your life.

Enjoy!

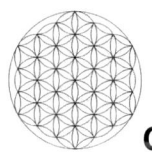

CHAPTER 5 SUMMARY

- Pushing beyond the point where you need to stop locks you into a pattern of boom and bust

- Yet you may feel unable to make a different choice - to put your recovery first

- Self-awareness is the first step to freeing yourself from this damaging pattern

- STOP before the battery dims – bank before you spend

ACTIONS

- Are you 'Taking Time'? If not, why not?

- Become aware of when you over-ride messages from your body

- Begin a daily diary to discover where you are using/losing energy

- Practice changing a negative reaction into a positive response

Chapter 6

Choices

In the last chapter you explored the pattern of boom and bust. When I ask the groups, 'What's driving your choice to push yourself too hard?' their responses include:

- *It's about reacting to other people's criticism, expectations, targets (echoed by many)*
- *what other people think of me matters*
- *other people don't understand*
- *it's to do with a sense of duty*
- *I guess I'm trying to be all things to all people*
- *It's what other people want of me*
- *feeling guilty, being guilty, drives my decisions*
- *I feel responsible for others*
- *It's about a feeling of self-achievement*
- *I need to feel in control (echoed several times)*
- *self criticism - am I being lazy?*
- *my G.P says I'm imagining I can't do things*
- *I've high expectations of myself*
- *I can't leave something that needs doing*

- *I don't want to be beaten*
- *I'm a perfectionist*
- *I'm trying to ignore/deny it (the illness)*
- *I want to feel normal*
- *I guess it's a habit - it's how I've always been*
- *my subconscious takes over; it's automatic*
- *I don't know why*

Take a good look at this list. How many are driven by other people's expectations or reactions? The first eight definitely, but most do in one way or another. Take *'I've high expectations of myself'* and *'I'm a perfectionist'*. It's likely these come from a desire to please.

Important - Whatever is behind your habit of pushing yourself too hard and getting locked into a pattern of boom and bust, don't use this awareness to criticise yourself.

Why? Because being hard on yourself never achieves anything, particularly when you're not making a conscious choice**.** The force of habit, the result of years of responding in a certain way, is making your choices for you. And without this course, it would carry on doing just that. But now you have the tools to replace old, unhelpful habits with new ones that support healing. Try shifting the emphasis:

- from *reacting* to others' expectations
- to *responding*, considering your own needs.

Choose to support your health and well-being by:

- listening and responding to your body instead of fighting and reacting to it
- trusting your body to know what it needs
- releasing old emotional patterns that are hampering your body's attempts to heal

How can you do this?

Take Out The Magnifying Glass

- take a close look at the choices you're making through a lens of extreme self care
- what would a compassionate friend say about those choices?
- when those choices aren't the most loving ones ask, 'what habit or pattern caused me to make that choice?'
- take a fresh look at the thoughts that lie beneath those habits or patterns
- do they make sense?
- if not, replace them with more loving, caring thoughts
- so you can make more caring choices
- that will support your body as it heals

A word about change.

Habit is such a strong force that many of your reactions will be automatic. (You'll take the same route despite reminding yourself about the road works) Most of the time this is okay. Thinking about every action would consume far too much of your time and energy. But habit can have its downside - particularly when it stops you from responding to your needs.

Unfortunately force of habit is such a part of you that when you first make a conscious decision to respond differently to a situation or a person, the habit may resist like crazy. It might feel completely wrong to do this. Perhaps the easiest way to describe it is to talk about 'the devil you know'. Familiarity has a strong pull, even if it's pulling you in the wrong direction.

Responding differently may seem to make things worse. This is because the thoughts you're changing have been buried for so long you haven't realised how negative they are. Suddenly it's almost as though you can't see anything else. And things can feel a whole lot worse.

Remind yourself that this feeling of 'wrongness' is simply change taking place. All the negativity that has been draining your energy for so long is on the way out.

Habit will resist the changes you're making, but try not to use up valuable energy resisting this resistance! Simply notice resistance is there and say to yourself, *'this is just change happening, and that's all right'*.

WHO AM I?

Your best friend or greatest enemy, I am your greatest companion. I am your greatest helper or your heaviest burden. I will push you onwards or drag you down to failure. I am completely at your command.

Half the things you do, you might as well turn over to me and I'll do them quickly and correctly. I'm easily managed, but you must be firm with me. Show me exactly how you want something done and, after a few lessons, I'll do it automatically. I'm the servant of all great men and, alas, of all failures as well.

Those who are great, I have made great. Those who are failures, I have made failures. I work with the precision of a scientist and the passion of a patriot. You may run me for profit or run me for ruin; it makes no difference to me.

Take me, train me, be firm with me and I will put the world at your feet - but be easy with me and I'll destroy you.

Who am I? I am Habit!

The key is for you to control me – not let me control you!   Anon

It takes practice to create positive new habits.

Catch yourself when you react automatically and either reverse the decision there and then or make a note to respond differently next time.

Catching your automatic responses.

How do you respond when someone says, 'can I help?'

- 'I'm fine thanks'
  or
- 'thank you, that would be great'

How easy is it for you to accept help? If your automatic reaction is, '*I'm fine,*' find a quiet, comfortable spot, **'Take Five'**… and explore your thoughts.

Do this now.

Are you fine? Possibly not. So why did you say you are? We'll look at this in the next chapter but for now, jot down any thoughts that are making it difficult for you to accept help when it's offered.

The more you practise the techniques covered in this course, the easier it becomes to make the positive choices that will bring about the most amazing changes in your life. Key to this is the will, for now, to make the quality of your life your absolute priority.

Within the practical constraints you cannot change, ask yourself:

- ➡ am I willing to focus on my Self?
- ➡ am I willing to make the quality of my life my top priority?

What you focus on is strengthened.

If you focus on illness it will dominate everything. It doesn't have to. We're going to shift the focus to the unique person that you are, relegating illness to something you manage with love and care but which no longer dominates your life.

Setting aside the impact illness has on your life, consider:

- ➡ what are your hopes and dreams?

- ➡ what brings you joy and satisfaction?

- ➡ what is your life purpose?

Give some time to these questions, they're fundamental to your recovery.

What direction do *you* want to take in *your* life? Regardless of the hopes and expectations of others, what gives your life meaning?

'Take Five', and allow yourself to dream - and dream big. Make it a multi-coloured, anything-goes dream.

Has your negative tape started up?:

- *what's the point, I'll never be able to do what I want to do*

- *how can I travel the world; go back to work; be a full-time mum; launch my own business; become creative... feeling like this?*

Press the pause button. **Give yourself permission to set these thoughts to one side then continue to dream.** Imagine you are free to be who you truly want to be and allow a seed of possibility to germinate.

Imagine a mosaic, a work of art created from the shattered pieces of other shapes, other forms. They may be unrecognisable as they once were but they've been re-created in a new, even more beautiful form.

Your previous life may have shattered, but instead of gluing the pieces back into something liable to break again, why not create a new mosaic, a new life. The choice is yours.

There'll be pieces from your previous life you'll want to keep, but fresh ones will also be needed to complete your new mosaic.

Creating Your New Life Mosaic

To create your new life mosaic, answer the following in as much detail as you can:

- what are your secret hopes and dreams?

- what fires your imagination?

- what fills you with enthusiasm?

- think back to childhood days - what were your ambitions then?

- complete the sentence, 'I've always wanted to...'

- what have you always secretly thought you'd be good at but not tried because of fear of criticism or ridicule?

As soon as any objections start to play on your internal tape turn down the volume and carry on dreaming. Find as many answers as you can to each of the questions. Write them in your journal, both now and as thoughts occur to you over the next few days and weeks. These are the pieces that will create your new life mosaic.

And finally...

During the next week make sure that you 'Take Time' for yourself ensuring your choice is completely enjoyable, easily within your reach and a treat.

Enjoy!

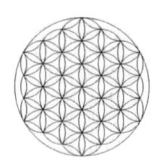

CHAPTER 6 SUMMARY

→ Are the expectations of others causing you to make inappropriate choices for yourself?

→ Use 'The Magnifying Glass' to become aware of those choices

→ Replace unhelpful choices with ones that support your health and well-being

→ Developing new, positive habits takes practice and a willingness to focus on your quality of life

→ What you focus on is strengthened - shift your focus from the illness to the unique person that you are

ACTIONS

→ Write about your hopes and dreams, your life purpose

→ Find the pieces for your new life mosaic

→ Continue 'Taking Time'

Chapter 7

Time for some T.L.C.

In the last chapter you explored how other people's expectations and reactions can prevent you, *often unknowingly*, from making the kindest choices for yourself. And you reflected on how habit - ingrained and automatic ways of thinking, feeling and reacting - can make it difficult to change.

As a child you became accustomed to reacting in a certain way in certain situations; not a problem when life is going fine but when you hit a challenge the old programming can cause you to come unstuck.

It's time to:

- become aware of any automatic reactions acquired during your childhood
- and release any that are undermining your recovery

How can you do this?

By catching your automatic reactions and consciously making a different choice about how to think, feel and respond.

Make this different choice a more loving, caring, considerate choice; a choice that meets your needs, not one based on the habits of the wonderful people who nurtured you to the best of their ability but who may have passed on unhelpful automatic reactions learnt from their parents.

Explore your family patterns

- were your parents or carers ever ill?
- how did they respond to illness – theirs or yours?
- how good were they at taking care of their own needs?

When I do this activity in the groups some common responses are:

- *they hid illness (echoed by many)*
- *my mother battled on (again echoed by many)*
- *it was a matter of pride not to admit they were ill*
- *'don't complain' was our family motto*
- *mind over matter*

- *it'll pass*
- *think positive*
- *there was a degree of self neglect*
- *they felt a duty to be responsible for others*
- *they'd say, 'You'll be all right'*

Look at your own list. Do you recognise any of these in yourself? Make a note of them in your journal.

> ### Ask yourself, do I...
>
> - hide illness?
> - battle on?
> - not admit I'm ill?
> - think mind over matter?
> - neglect myself?

Now **'Take Five'**...
...and when you're relaxed, very gently become aware of any patterns that may be preventing you from responding to yourself with love, care, consideration and patience.

Do this now.

Jot down your responses and then read them back with one question in mind. Have I adopted family patterns without even realising it?

Check in with your internal tape. Is it playing some familiar objections, arguing with you or resisting this exercise in some other way?

Maybe you're thinking:

- *this is who I am, you can't muck about with someone's personality*
- *there's no time for me with two young children*
- *I'm no good at relaxing, I've got to be doing*

And that's fine. It's only an unconscious resistance to change. Ask yourself, *'what could I do differently?'*

> **Recall a time when your body said 'stop' but you didn't respond**
>
> - fill in all the details:
>   - what was happening?
>   - what did you actually do?
>   - how did you feel afterwards?
>
> - now close your eyes, replay the scene and picture yourself making a different choice
>
> - follow your innermost promptings - see yourself saying and doing what was necessary to meet your needs

Your internal tape may object:

- t*hat's not realistic, I'd never be able to do that*

Have the courage to stay with this scene where you've chosen to meet your own needs. Watch and listen.

- what are you saying?
- what are you doing?

Perhaps you're going somewhere to be alone, or asking someone to do something for you. Imagine that everyone does as you ask without question.

If your tape butts in here be aware of what it says but stay with the scene you've created. How does it feel to respond to your innermost needs?

Time for some T.L.C.

In the last exercise you practised shifting the emphasis from your thoughts, and the negative internal tape that was your default setting, to your innermost promptings. They've probably been asking you to pay attention to them for a long time.

Maybe you were aware of them the last time you **knew** you should stop doing something but couldn't, the old programming and patterns were just too strong.

You can change that programming and free yourself up to make better choices by adopting a policy of T.L.C.**,** tender loving care, for yourself at all times.

Practising T.L.C. is a vital step in shifting the focus from the illness to your Self.

Tender	= gentle, unpressurised, patient
Loving	= considerate, appreciative, accepting
Care	= supporting, enabling, protecting

How kind and gentle are you with yourself? Are you your own best friend offering considerate, supportive advice and help? Or is your critical internal tape more often to be heard saying something like:

- *you don't have to stop already do you?*
- *what's wrong with you for goodness sake?*
- *why bother if you can't see it through?*

You can change this tape.
We talked about awareness earlier. The next step is acceptance. Not submission, not defeat, but acceptance of the need for TLC because:

- life is as it is - just for the moment
- the way forward lies in responding to how things are, not denying or fighting that reality

What you resist persists. What you focus on is strengthened. By fighting something you can actually reinforce it, making it an overwhelming factor in your life - absorbing much needed energy.

The Fight Between Two Wolves

An elder Cherokee Native American was teaching his grandchildren about life. He said to them, 'A fight is going on inside me... it is a terrible fight and it is between two wolves.

One wolf represents fear, anger, envy, sorrow, regret, greed, arrogance, self-pity, guilt, resentment, inferiority, lies, false pride, superiority, and ego.

The other stands for joy, peace, love, hope, sharing, serenity, humility, kindness, benevolence, friendship, empathy, generosity, truth, compassion, and faith.

This same fight is going on inside you, and inside every other person, too.'

They thought about it for a minute and then one child asked his grandfather, 'Which wolf will win?'

The old Cherokee simply replied... 'The one you feed.'

You have a choice.

- to continue to resist and resent the illness, feeding your anger and frustration

- or to listen, accepting that this experience may have something valuable to offer, feeding hope and health

Giving up resistance and making a different choice will mean challenging beliefs you've held for a long time, beliefs that feel very much like the truth. But if you're willing to consider other ways of thinking about illness, then all things are possible.

Relax for a moment and 'Take Five'.

Then imagine a young girl with a broken leg. As she struggles and fails to walk across the room do you lay into her, tell her she's not trying hard enough, insist she walks without your helping hand, shout at her when she falls, watch as she drives herself to exhaustion because she thinks that will please you?

Imagine yourself as that child. What will help you most? Maybe consideration, understanding, a loving, helping hand, time, patience. **You can offer all these to yourself.** Instead of remaining caught up in anger and bitterness, become your own greatest supporter, feeding compassion and hope.

Practising T.L.C[5]

- say no to others unless it's an absolute yes
- spend time and energy on things that bring you joy
- release yourself from the sometimes overwhelming expectations of others
- be gentle, kind and patient with yourself
- treat yourself as you would someone you really loved
- never criticise yourself - criticism doesn't change anything
- accept yourself as you are and watch positive change happen
- praise yourself - acknowledge all you are doing
- listen and respond to your body instead of fighting, resisting or reacting to it
- **know you deserve all of this and more**

---

[5]Inspired by the work of Cheryl Richardson, Louise Hay, Susan Jeffers, Patricia Crane and others

After awareness and acceptance comes action.

You've been reading about the positive action that *you* can take *right now* to make a difference to your life. I'd like to change the emphasis and say... this course is about the positive *action* you can take right now that will make a difference to your life.

As the saying goes, actions speak louder than words. Without action nothing will change. Select an action from 'Practicing T.L.C.' remembering to stay alert for the reaction that habit will generate. In the groups, 'Say no unless it's an absolute yes' always provokes a debate.

- *dream on!*
- *how can I do that?*
- *tell that to the kids/my partner/the boss*

Look back at the passages exploring how you've become conditioned to respond to the expectations of others and give yourself permission to make a different choice. This week, make your Self your absolute priority. Chose a different thing from the T.L.C. list to practise each day.

- replace self criticism with self appreciation, acknowledging everything you *can* do
- congratulate yourself when each activity is done
- recognise the skills you have and write them up as though they are entries on your C.V.
- build in rewards for each time you recognise a bout of self criticism and manage to turn it around

I'm lucky enough to live near the sea and for me, the promise of half an hour on the beach works wonders.

Practise every T.L.C. suggestion until you have a whole new range of positive habits that are consciously and unconsciously supporting your healing.

And finally...

During the next week, take even more time, ensuring whatever you do is completely enjoyable, easily within your reach and an absolute treat.

Enjoy!

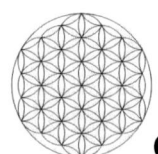

CHAPTER 7 SUMMARY

→ Are you unconsciously perpetuating family patterns surrounding illness?

→ Free yourself by responding to your inner promptings

→ What you resist persists - by fighting illness, you can reinforce it

→ Become your own best friend

→ Adopt a policy of T.L.C. at all times

ACTIONS

→ Identify family patterns surrounding illness

→ Imagine a situation when you ignored your inner promptings and picture yourself making a different choice

→ Offer yourself T.L.C. at every opportunity; you deserve it

Chapter 8

A Different Language

In the last chapter you looked at creating the best possible healing environment for your body by:

- becoming aware of your individual patterns and programming
- practising T.L.C. at every opportunity
- becoming aware of an inner guidance directing you to your best choices
- responding without allowing the mind to talk you out of what you intuitively know you need

Congratulate yourself!

Each time you catch a negative thought or pattern and make a different choice, congratulate yourself. Treat yourself to two films this week instead of one. Buy something you've been lusting after. Criticism never changed anything but rewards definitely work!

Reinforcing positive choices will make it easier to let go of negative ones. And your body will release tension and regain energy as you reduce inner conflict by being 'true to yourself'.

Remember Michelangelo:

> *Creating the David was easy; all I had to do was chip away all that was not David from the stone.*

A further word about change.

You may feel 'all at sea' for a while. This is normal; it's only change taking place. Imagine you're on a boat on the ocean. As familiar shores become more distant the sea gets rougher and you start to doubt the wisdom of your journey, particularly as you can't see your destination. But unless you let go of familiar shores and cross those turbulent seas you'll never reach the life you dream of.

A boat at sea is often off-course but by constantly making small adjustments in response to experience, it reaches its destination. Personal change is much the same. When you feel 'all at sea' keep making those small intuitive changes and you will get there.

Important
Ensure you have all the support you need, from yourself and others, to help you through this process. Imagine yourself in intensive care with your every need being met.

The only difference is that you are learning to meet your own emotional needs; *you*, the one person you know you can now depend on for support, love and care.

This intensive care involves harnessing all the resources available to support your immune system. Suggestions from the groups include:

- deep breathing
- banking, pacing, switching activities
- keeping occupied
- hydration - drinking enough water to help reduce brain fog
- diet - e.g. considering low sugar, wheat-free etc.
- therapies e.g. Reiki, Reflexology, Emotional Freedom Technique, Acupuncture, The Lightning Process
- stabilising sleep patterns
- relaxation - 'Take 5' and longer (20mins)
- meditation
- Tai Chi, yoga
- extreme self care and T.L.C.
- alone time, absolute quiet

These are just some of the things you can do to support your immune system and conserve or boost your energy. Combined with the techniques you're now using from this course, they have the power to transform your life.

Still feel stuck in a loop?

Maybe the boom and bust syndrome remains a part of your life and you're confused as to why. Maybe stress is still taking its toll.

Remember the Four Steps for reducing stress:

Step 1	'Take 5', breathe and relax.
Step 2	Identify the negative thoughts causing the stress. *'I'm never going to get my life back. What's the point?'*
Step 3	Remember; you can change these thoughts, they're a real pain anyway!
Step 4	And do it. Think positive. *'Following this course is making a difference.'*

We're now going to adapt these steps, particularly for situations where it's important to make choices based on your inner promptings, not the information being churned out on your well-worn tape. For example, when those promptings urge you to slow down or stop:

Step 1	'Take 5', breathe, relax and listen.
Step 2	Identify the negative thoughts pushing you to ignore those promptings: *'Why do anything if I have to stop already!'*
Step 4	Ask yourself, what patterns or expectations are driving these thoughts?
Step 4	Give yourself permission to make a different choice: *'If I stop now, I'll be able to do more tomorrow.'*

For example, I was driving home one day when I began to feel tired. I needed to stop. But my mind was arguing, *'it's only another 15 minutes, you can get home. You don't really feel that bad'.*

What patterns or expectations were driving those thoughts? I came up with the following possibilities:

- I was following a family pattern by pushing myself, by not showing weakness
- or by not feeling I could put my needs first
- I associated home with safety, security, sanctuary
- I was simply in a groove - I've started so I'll finish!

Having done this, I managed to pause the tape and make a different choice. I pulled into a Royal Horticultural Society car park, coincidentally the first opportunity I had to stop, to discover that they were having a free Open Day. I spent a wonderful half hour sitting in the gardens.

The one word that came out of this experience for me was... trust. I had to trust that my inner self knows best and that it will all work out if I respond to those whispered promptings. When I listened and responded, it worked out better than I could have planned.

- listen to your inner promptings
- become aware of the objections your mind raises
- assess those objections
- if appropriate, set them to one side
- and respond as your inner promptings urge

Why is it sometimes so difficult to do this?

Underlying beliefs can be very sticky. Imagine that you have an important meeting. Your first thought may be, '*I have to push myself. X is expecting me at four, I can't let him down. I don't have time to rest*'.

Having followed this course you now think: '*STOP. What's my body saying? Maybe that it's stressed and leaking energy far too fast. I'll pause, breathe, Take 5 and call X to say I'll be ten minutes late.*'

But maybe the tape simply picks up where it left off. '*Great theory but can't do it.*'

Why not? Why can't you do it? What underlying belief is stopping you from putting yourself first?

Have you ever been in the situation where someone bumps into you and <u>you</u> apologise? What's the underlying belief for this reaction? Maybe, '*whatever happens, it's my fault*'. Sadly many children grow up with this belief and it can be difficult to shake off as an adult.

Unconscious beliefs can influence all sorts of situations where they simply don't belong.

Returning to our example of the traffic jam, the negative thought might be: '*I'm going to be late, I'm letting everyone down, they'll be so mad*'.

What's the belief behind these thoughts? Perhaps that you'll lose their approval, shorthand for love, by letting them down; by not meeting their expectations of you. Take a deep breath. Would you instantly stop liking someone because there was too much traffic on the A38? Of course not.

Using a hefty dose of T.L.C., relax, change your thoughts and focus on the positives. *'They'll understand. I'll take this time to relax and listen to some music. I'm fine.'*

This course is like learning a new language.

Imagine yourself in a foreign country. You try to communicate in English because that's all you know. The result? You probably get by with a lot of gesticulation and guesswork but you're likely to feel increasingly isolated and frustrated, even angry or depressed - and unable to enjoy life to the full.

You now have a choice:

- to carry on as you are
  or
- to accept that your current learning is inappropriate and look for new solutions.

Having an illness is like being in a strange land where much of your previous learning is inappropriate.

Your circumstances have changed. The solutions your mind is offering no longer work. At an unconscious level they may be holding you back. Your mind may keep reminding you how great it was back in the good old days, constantly reinforcing your sense of loss. Disease will continue to be seen as a thief that has stolen everything you valued about your life.

There is another way of looking at disease.

That is to literally think of it as dis-ease, a sign that something is out of synch, out of harmony, telling you there's something to learn. It doesn't mean past learning is wrong, just inappropriate now. Your circumstances have changed, perhaps for a very good reason. Maybe there are benefits to be found in this situation. Maybe what appeared to be a disaster is actually an opportunity.

What thoughts are playing on your internal tape right now? In the groups some familiar ones are:

- *benefits! You must be crazy*
- *how can feeling like this possibly have anything good about it?*
- *do you think I want to feel like this?*
- *if you had the first idea of everything I've lost you wouldn't talk about benefits*

Perhaps you share some of the anger, sadness, frustration, fear and bitterness expressed here.

- anger because your needs, hopes, or expectations are not being met
- fear of feeling helpless, hopeless, disempowered

It's understandable if these feelings are dominating your life right now… but are they the best stepping stone to a new, happier life? Or are they draining you of energy and hampering your recovery?

Try detaching yourself from the powerful punch these feelings can generate. Become an observer. Set aside any judgements about whether they're right or wrong, good or bad. Simply:

- become **aware** of their presence
- **accept** that these feelings exist
- then take this opportunity for **action**
- and **practise making a different choice**

It's time to get curious. Set any resistance to one side and ask, '*if there were benefits to being ill, what might these be*?'

Look for the benefits

Thinking of illness as an opportunity not a disaster:

- what benefits has illness brought you?
- write your thoughts in your journal
- do this now

In the groups common responses include:

- time to take stock, smell the daisies, stand and stare
- time to re-think life, to plan a new life
- time to find out what really matters
- legitimate way to leave a stressful job or relationship
- permissible reason to ask for care from others
- opportunity to change direction

There are always positives to be found when you take a conscious decision to make a different choice.

What choice will you make? To constantly experience loss or to focus on opportunity?

Try it. Have a go at choosing to see how things are now as an opportunity not a disaster. What will the next few moments hold for you? Everything your negative tape has played over and over again or a new, positive experience?

Still not sure? What will you lose? Only the negative voice that's becoming a real pain anyway.

Create a private, comfortable space, 'Take Five' and then ask yourself...

- what one loving thing can I do for myself right now?

- let the answer come from within

- then make the choice to do that one thing for yourself

- decide when you will 'Take Time' to do it

- and make a commitment to do it

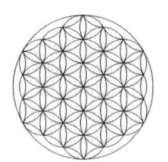

CHAPTER 8 SUMMARY

- Reconnect with the instinctive 'you' to find a reliable source of support and guidance

- Being 'all at sea' is okay, it's only change - ensure you're supported

- Release unhelpful family patterns surrounding illness

- Consider disease as dis-ease; indicating a need for change; opportunity not disaster

- What will the future hold? Everything your negative tape has replayed over and over or a new, more positive experience?

ACTIONS

- Using the Magnifying Glass and T.L.C., ask, 'am I making the best choices for myself?'

- Explore the possible benefits of illness

- Do one thing for yourself right now

Chapter 9

A Sense of Hope

At the end of the last chapter I asked you to do one loving thing for yourself. How did you get on?

If the answer's 'not too well' was there an element of 'should' about your choice rather than it being something you genuinely wanted to do?

Sometimes it's possible to become so identified with others that you take on their likes and dislikes without stopping to consider, 'is this what *I* want?' One way of discovering whether your choices are genuinely your own is to listen carefully to your language.

Without judging yourself in any way, reflect on when you use 'should', 'must', 'have to' when talking about the things you choose to do. The following exercise is based on suggestions made by Louise Hay, the author of several books on healing.[6] Use this exercise to discover what

---

[6] See 'You Can Heal Your Life' and 'The Power is Within You'

you've been doing for years that you never actually wanted to.

Are your choices based on what you feel is expected of you or to please a parent, partner, teacher or friend? Are they draining you of energy because your heart isn't in them?

The freedom to choose

This exercise is invaluable for identifying where your energies are being drained.

- how often do you use the word 'should'?

- just for a day, record each time you use the word 'should'

- at the end of the day look back over each incident

- ask yourself *'why should I?'*

- if you were completely free to choose, would you do the things you think you 'should' do?

- if not, why not?

- perhaps, *'because I don't want to!'*

Breaking the habit of meeting others' expectations may bring up all sorts of emotions; guilt is a common one. But you're not harming anyone else by putting yourself first once in a while. It's time to practise making a different choice, one that honours who you are.

There will probably be many things on your 'should' list that you still choose to do, helping others for example, but you avoid wasting energy on resistance and resentment once something becomes a choice. And when you decide not to do a 'should' you immediately release energy by saying no unless it's an absolute yes.

Simple.... or maybe not. You may be thinking, 'all this makes perfect sense but...'

- *I don't have a choice about lots of the things I do*
- *my sense of responsibility and duty over-ride everything else*
- *I can't let others down*

And the first thing you're going to tell yourself is - that's okay!

Because as your own best friend you know it's encouragement and reward that supports change, not criticism.

There's a familiar pattern with this illness. You get an initial burst of energy when you start something but then things rapidly go downhill. This is the boom and bust situation we looked at earlier. As the downhill plummet continues you know you're not listening to your body but something, maybe guilt, fear or frustration, drives you on and you're unable to make a different choice.

Whatever family patterns or habits are driving your choices, it's vital to establish the truth. Dr Darrel Ho-Yen, in his book *Better Recovery From Viral Illness* outlines some simple rules to conserve energy and then adds:

> *Although these rules are simple, for PVFS (post viral fatigue syndrome) patients they are extremely difficult as this involves facing the truth of their situation and taking appropriate action... When people lose their job, it can be a long time before they adjust to their reduced circumstances. Instead they continue to spend as before, hoping to be re-employed soon. The position is similar to PVFS patients, and, as with unemployment, those individuals who adjust best, do so early. Patients need to live within their budget (energy) now.*

If the truth is that you've exhausted your resources and need to stop immediately to prevent a relapse then:

- become aware of that truth
- acknowledge that truth
- respond to that truth

Remember to use **The Four Steps** to help you do this.

Step 1 Take Five, relax and listen when your inner promptings say *'slow down'* or *'stop'*.

Step 2	Identify the negative thoughts pushing you to override those promptings. *'What's the point if I have to stop already!'*
Step 3	Give yourself permission to make a different choice. *'If I stop now, I'll be able to do more tomorrow.'*
Step 4	And do it!

Most importantly, as well as highlighting where you've exhausted your resources it gives you the opportunity to ask, '*What is it about this particular activity that's draining my energy?*'

When your scores are low and you're ending each day feeling exhausted ask yourself:
- was my heart in everything I did?
- was I committed to it body and soul?

Take a fresh look at these familiar sayings. Read them literally. They highlight the importance of ensuring that your 'whole self' is behind everything you do; for your thoughts, words and actions to agree with each other and with your innermost promptings.

For example, do you become exhausted more quickly with some people than with others? Why is this? Does it happen more frequently at home or with acquaintances? If it happens more with acquaintances maybe it's just too much effort to make conversation with relative strangers. Or are you using valuable energy trying to relate to people you'd simply rather not be with?

If it happens more with someone closer perhaps there's a stress in the relationship that's literally depressing your system. Perhaps the dynamics are inhibiting you from being true to yourself, preventing you from speaking and acting truthfully.

> **What is the truth for you?**
>
> ➜ whenever you feel energy levels flagging
>
> ➜ take a fresh look at the circumstances
>
> ➜ ask yourself, *'what exactly am I tired of?'*

Answer this question with complete honesty. There may be things you'd rather not think about, but the stresses created by a difficult situation or relationship will still be experienced by your body. Even if you don't discuss your thoughts with others, have the courage to explore them honestly with yourself. What changes can you make to be who you truly are?

For example, you may be unhappy about a relationship you're in but for all sorts of reasons find it difficult to admit this, even to yourself. Or perhaps financial pressures mean you feel trapped in a career that you hate. Perhaps responsibilities for others are preventing you from living your own life. Do you choose not to look too closely at some aspects of your life? Do you sacrifice truth for fear of the consequences?

Important.

Exploring these issues may expose inner conflicts. Don't struggle with difficult issues alone. Remember to support yourself during this period of intensive care. Seek the help of trusted friends or a professional counsellor and build in as much T.L.C. as you can.

Emotional issues are rarely clear cut. You may doubt yourself and struggle to know what the truth is. When you feel uncertain try the following.

> **When you become aware of a conflict 'on the one hand this… on the other…'**
>
> - picture yourself taking each option in as much detail as you can
> - explore how your body feels with each option – relaxed or stressed?
> - does the relaxed option tie in with your inner promptings or intuition?
> - what is preventing you taking this option? Note how your internal tape, may be over-riding your inner promptings

There's a saying: **The truth is like a compass. It shows the way you want and need to go.**

If you choose not to explore what, besides illness, is causing imbalance and disharmony in your life, and do something about it, your body may continue to react with symptoms.

> **What changes do you need to make?**
>
> When you feel the battery dimming ask yourself:
>
> ➨ do I need to do less?
> **or**
> ➨ do I need to change what I am saying and doing so that my words and actions reflect the real me?

When your thoughts, words and deeds reflect your innermost self it can be like discovering a clear road ahead of you. Suddenly, instead of your life being a frustrating series of stops and starts it begins to flow and your way forward is clear.

A different kind of energy.

You'll discover a different kind of energy. Not the forced, adrenaline charge that gets you through a special event and leaves you exhausted, but a core energy that's constant. Becoming aware of, and responding to, the authentic 'you' recharges your battery naturally. And you'll find that your body begins to hold its charge instead of needing hours, days or weeks to recover.

It really is your choice.

This is the point where instead of saying, 'this course makes such good sense but…' and continuing to **react** to circumstances… you decide to make a different choice; to listen to your body, to **respond**.

- by saying STOP
- by fading out the negative voice on your internal tape
- by knowing that the uncomfortable emotions change produces, will fade
- by trusting your inner promptings
- by knowing this opens the door to a new sense of hope and possibility

Remember:

- if you always do what you always did
- you'll always get what you always got

Take time to reconnect with the real 'you'.

Read the following exercise and then make yourself comfortable somewhere you'll be undisturbed for at least twenty minutes. Close your eyes and create these pictures for yourself.

Visualise your Perfect Day

Take five and then...

imagine waking at the dawn of your perfect day
where are you?
perhaps on a tropical island
feeling the warm balmy air against your cheek

just now you are anywhere you want to be

look around at this wonderful place
what's so good about it?
maybe the absence of something
maybe the presence of something

in this moment anything is possible

all your hopes and dreams reveal themselves
what is your heart's desire?

what do you wish for yourself?
paint a picture of your wish in your mind
use all of your senses to bring that wish to life
give it colour, sound, light, sensation

see yourself living that wish
how do you feel as you live your wish?
give yourself permission to enjoy those feelings

this is your life
to live as you wish
you deserve it

if there's someone with you, see them delight
in your happiness

let your happiness be infectious
this is your perfect day

you are completely safe
completely loved
completely free to be yourself

this is who you truly are

stay with these feelings for as long as you
wish then slowly become aware of the room
around you, your body, sounds in and
outside, and without any rush at all, open
your eyes

decide on one step that you can take right
now towards your dream

And finally, 'Take Time' to build this step into your week, ensuring whatever you do is:

- something you enjoy
- easily within your reach
- and a treat

This is **your life** for you to live.

Enjoy!

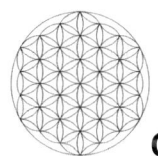

CHAPTER 9 SUMMARY

- Did you 'Take Time'? If not, was it a 'should' rather than something you genuinely wanted?

- Acknowledge the truth and make a different choice - instead of reacting, chose to listen to your body, to respond

- Finding this difficult? What underlying belief is preventing you from positive choices?

- This is your life to live as you wish - you deserve it

ACTIONS

- Complete the 'The Freedom to Choose' exercise

- What is the truth for you?

- Ask 'What am I tired of? Do I need to do less or change what I'm doing to reflect the real me?'

- Imagine your perfect day

Chapter 10

Rediscovering Your Self

In a previous chapter you considered the possibility that illness has benefits. Maybe becoming ill has:

- removed you from a pressurised situation
- given you much needed time - or time out
- enabled you to rest and take care of yourself
- provided you with a justifiable reason to say no
- made it okay to ask for care and consideration

All very positive benefits, even if your internal tape is making all sorts of judgements about illness being an unacceptable way of achieving them. You don't need to go there. Things are as they are for the moment. It's what happens now that's important.

The next step - making illness redundant.

The next step in recovering a life worth living is to make illness redundant. You do this by recognising the benefits it offers and finding another way of maintaining those benefits. It's time to make a commitment - that you will remain aware of and respond to your needs for the rest of your life.

Is your internal tape rewinding? *'Back to being selfish!'* Remind yourself right now of the enormous difference between selfishness at another's expense and self-care.

'Love one another as you love yourself' is a well-known dictum. But how many of us either forget or are unable to love ourselves? Yet without knowing how to love and care for yourself, truly loving and caring for others is impossible.

Here's another great benefit of your illness. In practising T.L.C. and focusing on your own self-care, you put in place the building blocks to be able to offer far more to others.

How do you create a new habit of caring for your Self?

By making this course an essential part of your life - not something you do for a week or two but that gets lost as life takes over again. With practise you'll find it increasingly easy to:

- fade out the old, inappropriate, internal tape
- release old habits
- quieten your mind
- become aware of your inner promptings
- listen
- and respond

> **Understanding brings growth
> but change needs action**
>
> ➜ look back over the exercises we've covered
>
> ➜ tick those you have actually practised
>
> ➜ maybe all of them, maybe none
>
> ➜ be honest with yourself

Changing habitual, negative reactions into positive, nurturing responses that will transform your life takes practice.

Have you ever bought a language book, skipped some of the exercises, rushed to the end, put it on the bookshelf and then been frustrated when you couldn't make yourself understood on your next holiday?

The language your mind is comfortable with has developed over your lifetime. To replace this takes practice and can feel like hard work when energy is in short supply. Recognise and accept your feelings, remind yourself of the consequences of not changing, and then focus on the new opportunities these changes will bring.

Also, be aware of something else that may be

influencing you - a very natural wish for someone else to provide the care you long for. Perhaps this illness is meeting that need. And that's absolutely fine. It's important not to criticise yourself for any of your choices. Equally, you may decide to make new choices because of the growing possibility that you can provide that care for yourself.

> **Changing habits**
>
> - look back over the exercises in this course
>
> - choose one thing from each - e.g. to be gentle, kind and patient with yourself (from the Practising T.L.C. exercise)
>
> - and make a commitment do it regularly
>
> - repetition is a great way to fade out old habits and establish new ones

Being authentically 'you' is another very effective way to create the best possible healing environment for your body.

How do you rediscover the 'real you'?

Have you heard of the saying, 'without fear or favour'? Train yourself to respond to people and circumstances without fear or favour and you'll rediscover your authentic self.

What does this mean?

Many of your thoughts and actions are determined by other people's expectations, by your **fear** of what they might think of you or your need to earn their approval or **favour**.

Your internal tape, that's now fading fast, was almost entirely made up of beliefs based on fear or favour. Practise deleting this tape, releasing any inappropriate need for the approval of others and replacing it with a deep respect for your Self. The astounding thing is that when we stop trying to be acceptable to others we almost always become more attractive to them!

My shorthand for this process is 'Holby City Authenticity'. Whenever I had this TV programme on and someone asked, *'are you watching this?'* my knee jerk reaction was to say, *'no, turn it over'.* I obviously was watching - and enjoying - it, so why did I say I wasn't? Looking back, I see an indignant 'inner me' jumping up and down wanting to know why I did that. I certainly hadn't responded authentically. Why not?

I needed to look beneath the words to the meaning I'd projected on to them. Picking up on negative tones and body language I heard, *'are you watching this?'* as *'you're not watching this rubbish are you?'* and felt an obligation to give way to someone else's preferences. Why? I slowly realised that I was acting from some deeply entrenched underlying beliefs:

- I had no right to have what I wanted
- Other people's judgements of right/wrong; good/bad were more important than mine

I was completely disempowered by a combination of fear and favour. I was unconsciously allowing someone else to determine my responses - which begged the question, who and why?

I focused on the voice playing on my internal tape and discovered an authoritarian voice from my childhood, my father. Because of my need to stay in his good books I'd compromised myself, or my Self, to meet his expectations. And thirty years later I was still responding in the same way, in situations where this pattern simply didn't belong!

This realisation gave me back my voice. It took practice and conscious awareness to make a change but, using the technique described in chapter eight of recreating the situation and then imagining a different response, the next time someone asked, *'are you watching this?'* I was able to say, *'yes, I am'*. Such a simple, but previously impossible, change was amazingly empowering and energising. Something shifted inside, like a dam suddenly giving way. My energy, the real me, was now free to flow.

> **Practise empowering yourself**
>
> ➜ think of a situation where you didn't act authentically
>
> ➜ rehearse a different 'true to yourself' response
>
> ➜ have a go at responding this way next time

A further word about change:

Changes you make as you follow this course may come as a surprise to those around you. The way you respond to others has developed over years. Present relationships may reflect familiar patterns from your early life, patterns you are now releasing in favour of more authentic ones. Changing your responses may create tension.

Do all you can to acknowledge the impact this process may have on those around you. Invite your loved ones to support you in the positive changes you are making, reassuring them that exploring your personal hopes and dreams does not have to be seen as a threat.

Considering and responding to the needs of others is a vital part of any relationship but make sure that any compromises you make are out of choice, moving from 'I should' to 'I could'. What you actually do may not change but there's a world of difference between an unconscious reaction and a conscious response.

An unconscious reaction might be to resent having to care for an elderly parent. Making a conscious choice to either offer care or find alternatives removes the hook. You may still be caring, but as a separate individual who has made that choice, not as someone bound by old emotional patterns to do what is expected of you.

Feeling overwhelmed? Or excited? The good news is it doesn't matter!

Understanding helps but it's what you do that matters. And the most important thing you can do right now is to spend more of your available energy on nurturing yourself. If necessary, sacrifice practical demands in favour of activities that are:

- completely enjoyable
- easily within your reach
- and a treat

Practise 'Taking Time' even more frequently, constantly reviewing and changing your choices to meet your changing needs.

Enjoy!

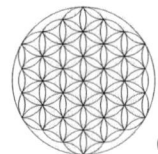

CHAPTER 10 SUMMARY

- Make illness redundant - recognise and respond to your own needs

- Illness can reflect dis-ease, inner conflict caused by unconsciously failing to respond to your true feelings

- Respond to others without fear or favour and rediscover your authentic self

- Being authentic recharges your battery naturally moment by moment

ACTIONS

- Write about the benefits illness offers you

- Do one thing from each exercise regularly

- Rehearse 'true to yourself' responses

Chapter 11

A Picture of Health

The body retains a memory of perfect health.

During a long period of illness, this memory can be masked by ongoing symptoms. Your mind reacts with thoughts such as, *'I'll never get better. I can't do anything anymore',* locking you into a cycle of ill-health.

The exercises described in this course can help to free you from that cycle. By becoming aware of, and changing, your thoughts you send a positive message to your body, encouraging it to live, prompting it to remember its natural healthy state.

Reinforce this process by completing the following at every opportunity.

Picture yourself

➜ Take Five and then...

➜ picture yourself as a child, full of energy

➜ create an imaginary movie of yourself as that child with the energy to do whatever you wished

➜ use all your senses - feel the warmth of the sun on your face or a friend's hand in yours, hear the beat of the music, taste the oranges, smell the new mown grass

➜ play this movie frequently, feeling all that energy surging through your body

➜ see each cell in your body as a battery that is now, slowly but surely, being recharged

➜ visualise the level rising to the top

This exercise will help to build a reservoir of energy that's different from the adrenaline burst that keeps you going for a while but then plunges you into boom and bust and continuing ill health.

Encouraging your body to build a reservoir of energy, and then treating that energy as a precious resource to be enjoyed, spent wisely and added to frequently, is the road to recovery.

Your imagination is a powerful tool for change, especially when used with positive affirmations. An affirmation is a great way to replace the negative sound bites playing over and over on your internal tape with the positive thoughts you'd like to hear. And by consciously changing the tape, you can actually change your experience of life.

Remember the traffic jam? If you want to change the negative tape that automatically starts to play when you find yourself late - *'great! I'll never get the job now'* - choose a positive phrase, *'every moment holds a new opportunity for me'*, and repeat it frequently. This one simple technique can transform the way you think and feel about life and create a new, more positive, reality.

Remember the discovery that stress lies not in a situation itself but in your reaction to that situation? Well, it's the same for your experience of life. It's not *what* happens that decides how good you feel about your life, but *your response* to what happens.

When ten bystanders observe an event they'll give ten different accounts of what happened. You have the power to choose your interpretation of events.

Some affirmations you might want to try are:

- every cell in my body is functioning perfectly
- my body is in perfect balance

What's playing on your internal tape right now? Maybe:

- *but that just isn't true*
- *I don't have anything like the energy I need*
- *my body isn't functioning perfectly at all!*

Thank your mind for the feedback, and for creating the perfect opportunity to practise interrupting the cycle of:

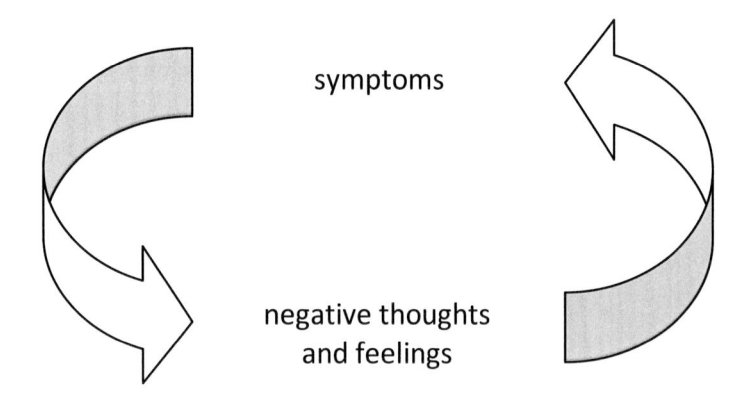

symptoms ⟲ negative thoughts and feelings

Write down the objections your mind came up with when you read the positive affirmations I suggested. Do this now.

Whatever you've written **is not the truth.**
- it may feel like the truth
- it may look like the truth
- your mind may have all sorts of justifications to prove it's the truth.

But it is only a thought. And you have a choice. To react to that thought, or to respond appropriately.

Look at the thought you've written down. See it as separate from you. Something you can choose whether or not to react to. For example if you wrote down, *'my body isn't functioning perfectly at all'*, pause... and take a good look at this thought. How does it make you feel? Not too good probably. Maybe you even feel physically worse focusing on this thought as though *thinking* about how bad you feel is actually *reinforcing* how bad you feel.

The good news is you can escape this cycle by becoming aware of and challenging those negative thoughts. So with the thought, *'my body isn't functioning perfectly at all'*, you can challenge it by remembering that much of your body is functioning just fine. You can then respond by taking some time out, booking a therapy or resting while supporting your body with a positive affirmation; for example, *'my body is healing'*. Make it your personal mantra, your response to every objection your mind throws up.

Take a good, uncritical look at this thought. *'My body is healing.'* How does it make you feel? Better?

Maybe your mind is saying something like, *'I'd feel better still if only it were true'*. You've come so far you can afford to be kind to your mind. It's been stuck in this loop for a long time. You now know how powerful habits and family patterns can be in programming your mind to react in this way.

Be gentle but firm as you guide your mind out of this negative loop and towards a new, more positive pathway. It may take some persuading but with practice it *will* start to believe you rather than vice versa! Your road to recovery can then look like this:

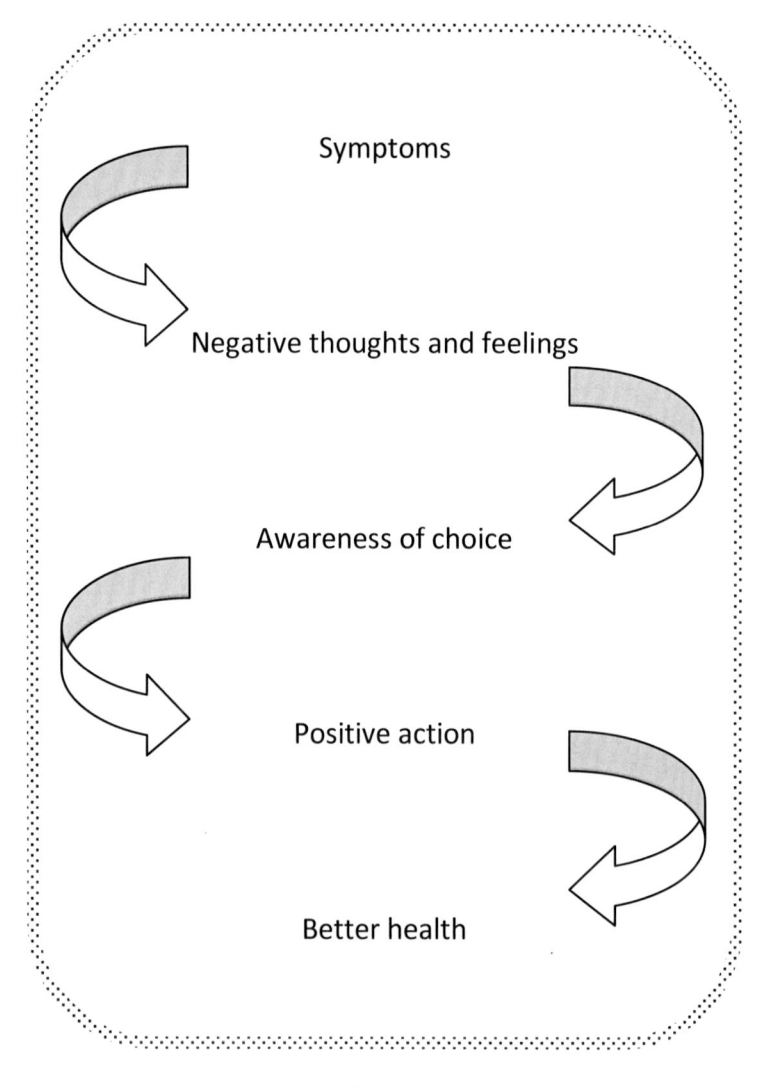

Symptoms

Negative thoughts and feelings

Awareness of choice

Positive action

Better health

Final thoughts.

At the beginning of this course I introduced you to the idea that your body has an amazing ability to self-heal, given the right conditions. I have provided you with the tools to identify and create those conditions for yourself.

This kind of change doesn't come from outside, from the actions of others or a change in circumstances. It comes from within. The emphasis is on **you,** on the positive, effective action **you** can take **right now** to make a difference to your life.

And it all comes down to the choices you make moment by moment. Remember:

when you become aware of your thoughts

⇩

you can begin to change those thoughts

⇩

and make different choices

⇩

to reduce stress

⇩

and support recovery

Choose to listen and respond to your body instead of fighting and reacting against it.

Choose to build a reservoir of energy by avoiding boom and bust and rediscovering the true 'you'.

Choose to relegate the illness to something you manage with love and care but which no longer has the power to dominate your life.

As you continue along your road to recovery...

Make a positive choice to support your health and well-being by 'Taking Time' every day, **realising that this is no longer a treat but an essential part of your life**. Not the life you had before, but a new one full of hope, opportunity, promise and health.

Enjoy!

Without referring back, answer the following

Circle the number that reflects how much you feel in control of your life. (Where 1 = not at all in control and 10 = completely in control)

1   2   3   4   5   6   7   8   9   10

Circle the number that reflects how much choice you feel you have in your life. (Where 1 = no choice, and 10 = complete choice)

1   2   3   4   5   6   7   8   9   10

Circle the number that reflects your sense of opportunity in life (Where 1 = I see no new opportunities, and 10 = my life is filled with new opportunities)

1   2   3   4   5   6   7   8   9   10

Now compare these scores with those you gave at the beginning of the course.

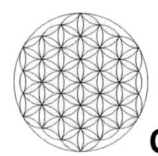

CHAPTER 11 SUMMARY

- Use the exercises from this course to free yourself from the cycle of: symptoms ⇨ negative thoughts and feelings ⇨ symptoms

- Send a positive 'live' message to your body

- Use imagination and affirmations to build a reservoir of energy, a precious resource to be spent wisely and added to frequently

- 'Take Time' every day, no longer a treat but an essential part of your life

- What other life have you yet to discover?

ACTIONS

- Complete the 'Picture Yourself' exercise as often as possible

- Practise using positive affirmations

- Compare your scores with those from the beginning of the course

- Enjoy your life

Postscript

My Story

I suffered from post-viral fatigue syndrome for over ten years, stuck in a vicious cycle of worsening symptoms. Then I made a life-changing discovery: for years I had unknowingly been undermining my body's amazing ability to self-heal.

This discovery was the key to breaking that cycle. Suddenly the way forward was filled with a sense of possibility not further loss. Drawing on insights gained during my professional career as a life coach and tutor of self management courses for the chronically ill, I evolved and ran courses to help others chart their own path to recovery.

Through this book, you can discover this process for yourself. This kind of change doesn't come from outside, from the actions of others or a change in circumstances. It comes from within. The emphasis is on you, on the positive, effective action you can take right now to make a difference to your life.

This is my story of illness and recovery.

Twenty years ago I took a break from my professional career to become the director of a company offering activity holidays. The company, alongside a lively family and social life, demanded immense amounts of time and energy. I was also physically active and thought nothing of heading out for a fourteen mile walk up and down the most tortuous stretches of the coastal footpath.

As far as I could then see it, my life was great. But there's another perspective on my life that I was either unwilling or unable to acknowledge. Looking back, I now see a flurry of activity that, like a centrifugal force, temporarily held everything together around a hollow core. Instead of purpose and joy emanating from a deep and authentic sense of myself it was a hit and miss by-product of an overly active lifestyle. Caught up in 'doing' enabled me to avoid acknowledging my hollow core and the pain it brought me.

This was a fundamentally unsustainable way of life. My body knew it but I couldn't see it. At that time, the unconscious programming driving my choices was so strong that I couldn't have acted any differently. I was locked into a pattern of denying myself to meet the expectations of others, a habit I'd acquired as a young child to gain the love of those around me.

Sadly it was never going to work because they'd never received the unconditional love that would have enabled them to wrap their arms around me, look unselfconsciously into my eyes and affirm the truth; that I was perfectly loveable, loving and loved.

I was as far removed from the person I essentially am

as it was possible to get. It was as though I had strayed into a fairground and found myself in a Hall of Mirrors where every way I turned I was a different shape. None felt comfortable or right but I couldn't tell why. I had totally lost sight of who I truly was.

Everything was now in place for me to discover my road to recovery.

One spring, the usual promise of renewal and regeneration was completely absent from my life. I was reeling from illness, divorce and bereavement. Looking back, it's no surprise that, when a persistent virus came along, my immune system gave up the ghost.

Liz Welch, a cranio-sacral therapist, has written, *'through my training in trauma work, I have come to realise that when a person becomes ill with M.E., it is likely that they already have some unresolved trauma in their system, which predisposes them to be overwhelmed by a further traumatic event, an accident or perhaps a virus infection.'*

For me this was absolutely the case. Six months later I was diagnosed with post-viral fatigue syndrome.

I sank into a black hole of loss and depression. Finding a local group helped me to a place where I could begin to benefit from various therapies and reach some kind of reconciliation with this illness. But I still had a lot to learn. In a desperate attempt to reclaim the life I'd lost, I continued to fight my body, plunging it into a damaging cycle of boom and bust.

But my body kept trying to communicate something I'd

needed to know for a long time but sadly wasn't willing or able to hear. After too long spent wasting what little energy I had on resisting and resenting the illness, the penny finally dropped. Instead of reacting to my body I began responding to it. I began to listen.

I began with the basics of relaxation and awareness and then took the time to ask, 'What is this illness all about? What is it I need to know? What changes do I need to make?'

To begin with my overactive, over-analysing mind supplied some very practical and often medical answers. 'It's a magnesium deficiency; fit the injections in between work and parents evening and you'll be fine.' Useful advice, but not the whole story and not enough to set me on the road to recovery.

So I decided to set this information aside and create a peaceful space for a different response. It didn't always come as words; sometimes it was an instinctive knowing or sudden realisation of what was needed. But all led me to one conclusion. It was time to take care of myself. I had driven myself too hard for too long.

I promised to pay attention to my Self.

The first and most difficult step was to stop work. The worries were immense. I was a single parent. How could I pay the mortgage and support my son? These were desperate times. But as I now know, when circumstances force us onto our knees that's exactly when life, God, universal intelligence, however you describe the force that unites us, can find a way through our defences and begin to guide and support us.

Using the techniques described in this book, I began to see things differently; to understand that the thoughts and beliefs driving my actions were misplaced. To change my life I simply had to change the way I thought about myself and my circumstances - although simply may not be the right word!

It's taken time, constant awareness and practice to shed the person I thought I was and begin to rediscover the person I am. Michelangelo's quote helped:

> *Creating the David was easy - all I had to do was chip away all that was not David from the stone.*

Letting go of past emotional habits and ways of thinking that were undermining my health has been a challenging but wonderful process. As I've taken each step to rediscover the essential 'me', my body has breathed a sigh of relief and my health has improved.

Through focusing on my body as a wonderful feedback device that tells me everything I need to know, as long as I take the time to ask and to listen, I've discovered a new choice. Instead of reacting with anger or fear I can respond with love and care. Now all the excellent therapies available to me make a difference because my choices support rather than undermine my body's ability to heal.

My health improved significantly and I returned to my professional career, working full time again until it became a choice, my choice, to opt for part-time. There's no sense of reclaiming my previous life though. This is a new life, a better life, underpinned by ways of thinking and being that constantly support rather than undermine my health and well-being.

For me illness was literally a blessing in disguise. It was the crisis I needed to make me wake up and take responsibility, meaning the ability to respond, for my Self. Please take time, all the time you need, to set yourself on course for recovery.'

Pamela Vass

March 2013

'On Course for Recovery'
Tutored courses

Introductory courses and workshops based on this text and led by Pamela are available for groups.

For further information or to order copies of this book see: www.boundstonebooks.co.uk

Suggested Reading

These are just some of the inspirational texts that are available on the subject of personal healing in the widest sense.

Better Recovery from Viral Illness – Dr Darrell Ho Yen
Creative Visualization – Shakti Gawain
End the Struggle and Dance with Life – Susan Jeffers
Feel the Fear and Do it Anyway – Susan Jeffers
Getting Well Again – O. Carl Simonton, Stephanie Matthews-Simonton, James L. Creighton
Heal Your Life – Louise Hay
Love, Medicine and Miracles – Bernie Siegel, M.D,
M.E., Post-Viral Fatigue Syndrome. How to Live With It – Dr Anne Macintyre
Ordering from the Cosmic Kitchen – Patricia J. Crane
Take Time for Your life - Cheryl Richardson
The Artist's Way – Julia Cameron
The Journey – Brandon Days
The Power is Within You – Louise Hay
The Power of Now – Eckhart Tolle
The Spontaneous Healing of Belief – Gregg Braden
The 10 Minute Life Coach – Fiona Harrold
Think and Heal - Professor Kurt Tepperwein
Quantum Healing – Deepak Chopra, M.D.
Why People Don't Heal and How They Can – Caroline Myss
When I Loved Myself Enough – Kim McMillen
Wide Awake – Erwin Raphael McManus

The Flower of Life

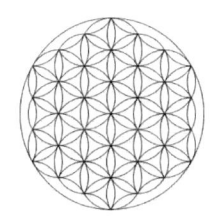

The Flower of Life is an ancient symbol reflecting the unity of life and the potential for emotional and physical healing from the heart. Through discovering the true Self, beyond all limiting thoughts and beliefs, we gain an immense sense of possibility, harmony and balance.